How Does She Do It?

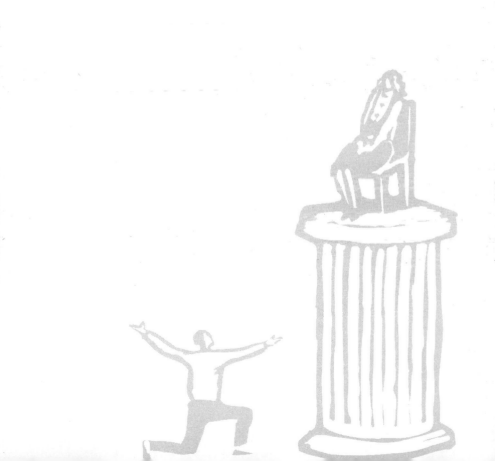

Also by Sheila Ellison

The Courage to Be a Single Mother
The Courage to Love Again
365 Days of Creative Play
365 Foods Kids Love to Eat
365 Games Babies Play
365 Games Toddlers Play
365 Afterschool Activities
365 Ways to Raise Great Kids

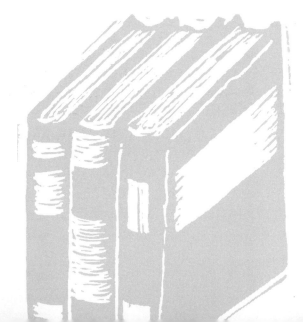

How Does She Do It?

101 LIFE LESSONS FROM ONE MOTHER TO ANOTHER

Sheila Ellison

HarperSanFrancisco
A Division of HarperCollins*Publishers*

HarperCollins books may be purchased for educational, business, or sales pro-
motional use. For information please write: Special Markets Department,
HarperCollins Publishers, Inc., 10 East 53rd Street, New York, NY 10022.

HarperCollins Web site: http://www.harpercollins.com

HarperCollins®, 🏭 ®, and HarperSanFrancisco™ are trademarks of HarperCollins
Publishers, Inc.

FIRST EDITION

Designed by Kris Tobiassen

Library of Congress Cataloging-in-Publication Data

Ellison, Sheila
    How does she do it? : 101 life lessons from one mother to another / Sheila
Ellison.—1st ed.
        p.   cm.
    ISBN 0–06–058370–3 (cloth)
    1. Mothers—Anecdotes. 2. Mothers—Quotations. I. Title.

HQ759.E465 2004
306.874'3—dc22   2003068596

04 05 06 07 08 RRD(H) 10 9 8 7 6 5 4 3 2 1

For Nancy Moshenrose Maley,
*my mother, who showed me with her encouragement, love,
creative tidbits, humor, and wisdom exactly how it's done.*

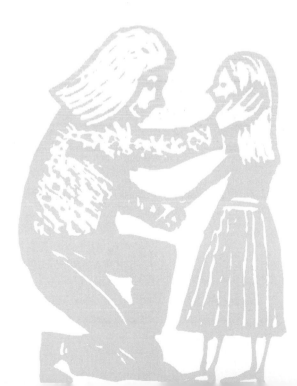

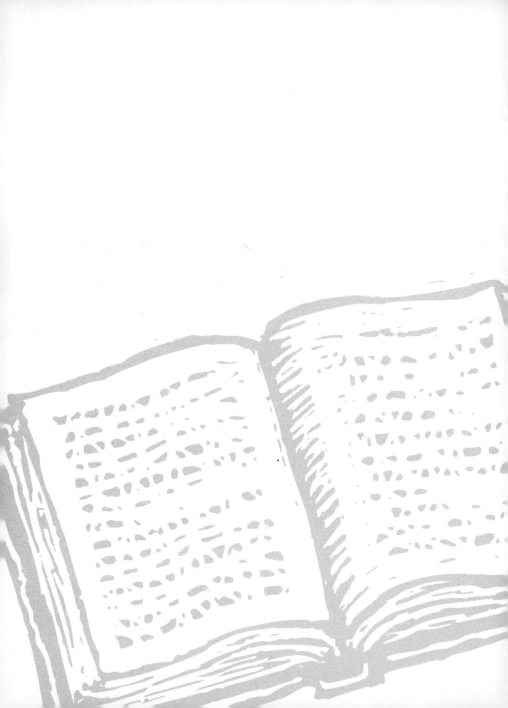

Contents

An Invitation

ello, fellow mother, this is your invitation to join me for a cup of tea. I know, there isn't time. You need to be multi-tasking—licking envelopes or changing diapers while we chat or you'll never fit all your daily tasks and responsibilities into the allotted time. Me too—I just returned from a meeting and have ten minutes before the kids arrive and the homework begins. But if I don't take five minutes for a break in my day, if only for a moment—I'll be bitter and irritated by nine—so please join me.

Pull up a chair, have a cookie. As mothers, we sometimes need reminding what all the homemaking, cooking, loving, working, and growing is for. I know because I forget myself—I get caught up in the day-to-day grind, with a list of things to do scrunched in my hand, feeling completely out of touch with the happiness I thought this mothering job would bring. I forget to shine a light now and then on the glorious success I am in all areas of my life—even on the most hectic days.

I try to remind my friends who are moms (and they do the same for me) that they are glorious successes—amazing, take-action, problem-solving, creative, compassionate women. We have learned our skills the hard way—through raising kids. We've triumphed over potty training, craft projects, bullies, broken hearts, driving lessons, and college applications—all while juggling our own lives.

On the following pages, you will find snapshots and excerpts from your own life. Don't worry: I haven't been looking through your window, eavesdropping on your most intimate conversations with girlfriends, or reading your diaries—but you may think I have. That's because we live remarkably similar lives as we try to raise great kids, have loving relationships, establish fulfilling careers, and still find time to grow into the women we want to be. But we have a tendency to lose our way. We focus on what isn't working instead of all the things we're doing well twenty-four hours a day. We may look at another mother and think, how does she do it? Well, here's the secret: we already know.

So please pull up a chair and give yourself a moment to get comfy as you settle in. I hope the following stories give you strength to face whatever this day may bring and help you to celebrate your monumental accomplishments as women and as mothers.

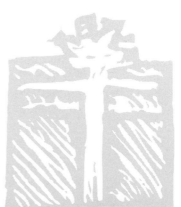

Celebrate Yourself

I'm tough, ambitious, and I know exactly what I want. If that makes me a bitch, okay.

—MADONNA

This year on my birthday I did something unusual. Instead of staying home and waiting for someone to plan some special event for me, I signed up for a gardening workshop for the entire day. I left before anyone asked me to make breakfast and returned to a dinner ready to be served!

At first I felt guilty, thinking my kids would be hurt if I chose to spend the day away from them. But with age I'm learning how to listen to my inner voice to determine what I *want*—and then to have the courage to make it happen. I used to sit back and hope that my children or husband would climb into my thoughts and figure out exactly how I'd like to celebrate my special day. I wanted them to demonstrate their ability to put my needs and wants first—like I do for them. Then at the end of the day, if they did not live up to my expectations, I felt unloved.

So this year when they asked what I wanted, I thought long and hard and gave them a specific request: I wanted my yard weeded. Smirks and frowns appeared. I was asking for their time instead of a trip to the mall for a quick and easy purchase. Of course, the kids had their excuses and planned events that prevented them from giving me what I asked for—although the lawn was mowed and some weeding had occurred. But this year I didn't care. I felt happy after spending the day learning about something I love.

My lesson this day was one I will remember. The little things in life that annoy, disappoint, hurt, or upset us don't seem so big or even worth considering when we've taken the time to nurture and care for ourselves.

Today I will do something that nurtures me.

2.

Laugh Now, Clean Up Later

Don't get your knickers in a knot. Nothing is solved and it just makes you walk funny.

—KATHRYN CARPENTER

One day when my son was still a baby, I came home to find him with bits of wet cement stuck to his clothes, skin, and diapers.

He'd gotten into the wheelbarrow where his dad was mixing cement to make a small walkway. Instead of capturing the hilarious sight of him on film, I immediately swooped in and cleaned him up—after cursing his father for not keeping a better eye on him.

As my children have grown up, I remember many an incident that, when I look back on it now, would have made *America's Funniest Home Videos* look boring. But instead of laughing or getting some perspective on the situation, I chose to assume the role of responsible adult.

Laughing, after all, would have given my kids the wrong idea. It would have been positive reinforcement for a negative behavior—according to all good parenting literature. The doll with the broken arm who got bandaged with my best silk scarf and the home movie I found where the boys were jumping from the high branches of the redwood tree onto the trampoline both make me laugh when I think about them now.

When I remember all the funny scenes, I am the one in the middle putting everything back together, teaching my kids what better choice they could make next time. Yet these are the scenes I remember most. They are the things the kids talk about around the dinner table for years afterward, laughing hysterically. I wish I could have laughed in the moment and cleaned up later.

Since my children continue to make unusual choices, there's still time to laugh first and clean up later! From now on, I will laugh for as long as I like, without worrying about what behavior I'm reinforcing. Then, when the time is right, I'll sit down like a good mom and explain the consequences.

I can learn to put my responsible adult self aside
and laugh in the moment.

3.

Forget the Spoonful of Sugar

It's not true that life is one damn thing after another; it is one damn thing over and over.

—EDNA ST. VINCENT MILLAY

Scattered' is the word I've always used to describe my life," said Sandy, the mother of two teens. "Nothing ever seems to be in order, I don't have time to keep my house clean, and most of the time I'm not sure where anything is. I don't exactly like my life this way; it's just the way it's turned out! But there are days when I dream of that scene from *Mary Poppins* where all the mess in the kids' room magically dances back into place!"

For most of us, having a clean, orderly, presentable home brings great satisfaction. We just don't have the time or energy to achieve it! It may be important, but in the scheme of our lives it seems to take a backseat to our everyday responsibilities. Maybe you've avoided your house's closets and drawers because there are so many—cleaning just one would make no difference whatsoever. Or perhaps you've experienced cleaning binges, devoting a day or two to the garage or your closet, just to find it a complete mess a month later—so why bother?

4.

"You Never Listen to Me"

Listening is a magnetic and strange thing, a creative
force. When we really listen to people there is an alternat-
ing current, and this recharges us so that we never get
tired of each other. We are constantly being re-created.

—BRENDA UELAND

G ood, consistent communication seems to be the key to
everything: lasting marriages, positive parenting, even
the training of pets! Most of us don't have a problem with the
talking part of the communication equation—where things
break down is on the listening end.

I once overheard a conversation between two twenty-four-
year-old men who had just hours earlier expressed to me their
frustration at not being able to create a lasting relationship. One
of them was advising the other, "You just need to keep asking
questions, nod your head, and pretend you're listening. That's all
women want—to get a chance to talk."

What they obviously hadn't figured out yet was that listening
can be a loving act that establishes intimacy. If you are just nodding and asking more questions without mixing in a bit of compassion, understanding, and interest, you are wasting your time.

Mothers in general are the best of listeners, yet sometimes a
child will say, "You never listen to me. You think you know me,

Yet most of us would admit that we love the feeling of being able to see our clothes and walk through our living room without tripping on piles. Our home reflects what we value—we want to feel happy and comfortable while enjoying it. So the question becomes, how can we achieve this with as little effort as possible? And how do we teach our children to organize and clean up after themselves?

In as little as thirty minutes a day, your entire life can become organized so that the word "scattered" no longer defines you. As always, organization begins with a list! Write the name of each room in your home you'd like to organize. Under the room, write the jobs that need to be done. Decide when you'd like to do your thirty-minute daily routine. Then, on day one, set your timer and start at the top of the list. *Stop* at thirty minutes. Entertain yourself with your favorite music or a book on tape. This technique works for kids too, but have them set their timers for ten minutes. They can organize their rooms, toy boxes, desks, the bathroom, or the yard! At the end of a few months you'll have made it through your list without having to set whole days aside for a major home overhaul!

When confronted with a messy, disorganized house, I will take care of it in manageable, short chunks of time.

but you don't." This is the time when it's most important to model great listening skills—so instead of defending yourself, use this opportunity to prove you know how to listen.

Respond with, "So you don't think I'm listening," and then encourage your child to talk. Hear what she says and then repeat it back to her in a different way until you are clear on what she means. If you actively listen in this way long enough, staying focused on what your child is saying instead of defending yourself or going off in a new direction, you will get to know what she really thinks or feels.

As mothers, we do more listening than anyone in the family, which means that our children and spouse see the example we set. If they fail to learn this listening technique, a little education on your part may produce compassionate, understanding, and interested communicators instead of a bunch of nodding heads.

Listening is an act of love.

5.

Stories We Tell Ourselves

Most of the shadows of this life are caused by our standing in our own sunshine.

—RALPH WALDO EMERSON

For the last few months I've been paying close attention to all of my negative thoughts," said Andrea. "I haven't tried to change or manipulate them; rather, I've approached this as a detective might, observing how my brain works. What I found was that I don't really have negative thoughts. In fact, my individual thoughts are pretty positive. Instead, I have entire stories I tell myself.

"I took a day to write down the stories as they drifted into my mind and was surprised by the frequency of these negative tidbits and the fact that many of the stories are ones I've been telling myself since I was a teenager! For example, when I wanted to pick up a book to read for an hour, the story in my head began, 'People who take breaks in the middle of the workday are lazy and will never accomplish their goals.' Later that day, when my husband asked what something had cost, the story continued, 'He is trying to control me by questioning my right to spend my own money.'

"These stories went on all day, and the scary thing was that I acted on them as if they were real—the truth of my life. As an experiment, I decided to catch each story in mid-track and ask myself relevant questions—like, when did I start to believe that relaxing was the definition of lazy? What if my husband was just curious about the cost and didn't care at all about what I spent?"

Pay attention today to the stories you tell yourself—about your love life, relationship, kids, parents, or friends. What career stories do you repeat when you're overlooked for a promotion or even given exactly what you've asked for? Look at the daily judgments you make and then try to figure out where and when the stories you now believe became a part of who you are.

"Once I understood that these stories were merely ideas that live in my head, I felt great relief," said Andrea. "It means they can be rewritten to suit the woman I am today, a woman who can choose to live and believe anything she wants. After all, they are my stories to begin with."

The stories I've told myself may not be true for me now—
I am the writer of new stories.

6.

Not All Children Are Created Equal

Likely as not, the child you can do least with will do the most to make you proud.

—MIGNON MCLAUGHLIN

Yesterday I struggled (and cried) over the realization that my kids are not created equal. Yes, I love them all the same beyond description, and I've made the effort to point out all of their individual and unique talents, but some of them have talents and skills that far surpass the others'. That's hard to explain to a kid—why he or she isn't nearly as good at something as a brother or sister. It is even more difficult if the child noticing this inequality has obvious disabilities.

I can usually come up with very creative solutions to every family issue, but this one has stumped me. I've been preparing for this since my son was diagnosed with high-functioning autism, building him up, pointing out all the ways he shines in the world.

But the truth is that he doesn't shine the way he wants to, and there isn't anything I can do to make it better. He has amazing strengths, like his ability to keep his room neat and clean, his love of animals, and his creative moviemaking skills—but those aren't the ones being valued out in the world.

He wants to be just like everyone else, scoring high on math tests, understanding basketball plays without having to study them, or talking without thinking. In his view of the world, he is the only one struggling while the rest of us sail through our lives with little to no effort. In some ways he's right. I tell him that his time will come, that things will get easier with practice. All he says is, "When?"

Sometimes we love with all our might and yet we still have to stand back and let life happen, admitting that we have no power to make it better for our children. To love another human being so much it hurts is life's greatest blessing. Being able to accept the lives our children are given can be a challenge. Helping them to see and accept themselves for the unique and loved persons they are is our job.

Today I will allow my children the dignity of their own struggles.

7.

The Compliment Cure

Children are likely to live up to what you believe of them.

—LADY BIRD JOHNSON

Given the fact that few of us have any real mothering training before our first baby is placed in our arms, raising kids is tantamount to conducting one experiment after another. My latest experiment is in the use of compliments. I collected data and found that for every one positive compliment I gave my children, I had made five to ten negative corrective comments.

My new plan was to try to catch the kids doing something right and then compliment them on their behavior, instead of pointing out the wrong. This is a complete reversal for me—I've always given compliments, but never with the intent to mold my kids' behavior.

So far the outcome has been promising. Instead of scolding them for forgetting to put their dishes in the dishwasher, I gave massive praise to the one child who actually carried an empty glass from his bedroom to the kitchen. Taking note, the other kids made the comment that it wasn't that big a deal. Why was I being so nice about a stupid glass?

But guess what? The next day I saw many dishes in the dishwasher—and I hadn't put them there! Children, no matter what age, blossom when you take the time to point out what they are doing right.

After a week of sleuthing for good behaviors, I'm a believer that better behavior is shaped more by positive compliments than when negative observation is used. We all want to please those we love, so get in the habit of pointing out really great things about your child every day. Catch him doing something good and watch what happens.

P.S. This works equally well on a spouse!

Today I will notice all the great things about my kids and let them know how special they are.

8.

"You Let Your Kid Do What?"

When I stopped seeing my mother with the eyes of a child, I saw the woman who helped me give birth to myself.

—NANCY FRIDAY

When my daughter attended her last high school prom, I had the pre-prom party. Over a chocolate-covered strawberry, I told one of the fathers that Wesley and a few friends had rented a hotel room in San Francisco. The man looked shocked. It was in this moment that I realized how much I trust my children. That isn't to say I expect them to go through life never getting into trouble and always making the right choices. Rather, over the past few years I've worked on the concept of letting go and believing that the hours spent teaching, modeling, advising, and loving my children will be enough to see them through.

Our children will not always live within sight, and they grow and change in ways we cannot control or even direct. I've struggled often with what choice to make, but in almost every situation I've been willing to listen to what they've wanted and tried to work within their plans. In return, I've been blessed with open communication—I know when there are drugs at a party, which of their friends is having sex, and when they are faced with serious problems or difficult choices.

We cannot make the actual choices for them. They will be confronted with temptations and opportunities we would like to ignore or pretend do not exist. I wanted to tell the father that his son was eighteen years old and that at some point all we can do is let go and believe that we've given our child the life skills he'll need to survive. But I kept eating my strawberry, having determined a long time ago that one of the fun aspects of parenting is the experimental nature of it all—each parent must embark on a life journey with his or her own child. Nobody has a map!

I will celebrate my children and give them the freedom they need to grow into themselves.

9.

The Joy of Lowered Expectations

The man who removes a mountain begins by carrying away small stones.

—CHINESE PROVERB

"Until about a year ago gardening used to be a deep love of mine," said Margaret, the mother of three boys. "It was on a Saturday in March, and I was decked out in a sun hat and rubber gloves as I tried desperately to save my perennials, which were being strangled by invasive weeds. I looked around the garden and felt completely overwhelmed. Even if I spent every weekend for the next three months elbow-deep in dirt, I could not keep up with the demands of my garden—so I peeled off my gloves, stomped resentfully into the house, made a cup of tea, and let my garden go.

"A year later I had a delightful conversation with a woman who loves to garden. We talked about how pretty blueberry bushes look in the fall with their colorful leaves, and the delicious, full taste of homegrown tomatoes. While we talked, something inside started screaming to get out—I wanted to go home and plant a vegetable garden. Knowing my history of setting high expectations and then feeling defeated when I couldn't reach them, I decided this would be a small vegetable patch."

So what had changed in Margaret that allowed her old passion to reenter her life with a more realistic vision? She let go of something she'd always loved because she was overwhelmed to the point that it no longer brought her joy. There are things we do in our lives that fill us up and make us feel more alive when we're doing them—gardening was like that for Margaret. Then there are times when what we love to do becomes something we must do, or something we're obsessed with doing, and it can become overwhelming. Which is how Margaret felt when she realized her expectations for her garden were more than she could manage. We need to be able to step back and ask ourselves, what feels good and what brings us joy right now? Then we need to be realistic in setting expectations—how much can we really cram into our lives, and how much can we take responsibility for, if the goal is to create a healthy mind and spirit?

If I lower my expectations, I will find more joy
in the ordinary corners of my life.

What It Means to Be Courageous

Laugh out loud, resist fear, take on a new challenge—find out what life has to offer by sticking out your neck.

—GABRIELLE REECE

This world can be a pretty scary place—especially for mothers. When I was in college, I was a youth director at a Catholic church in a high-crime area of Los Angeles. The kids told me daily about abusive parents, drug use, gang initiations, the prejudice they experienced, and the danger for me of going anywhere alone. I should have been afraid, but fear never crossed my mind—I was too full of youthful purpose.

A few years later my first child was born, and I found it impossible to make the same choices—I was afraid of things that had never scared me before. Once we've held a child in our arms, we look at the world differently. The reckless abandon of our youth and our belief that nothing can hurt us turn into all sorts of fears. Will I be a good enough mother? How do I keep my children safe from abduction, abuse, bullying, and sickness? What happens if I can't make enough money to buy groceries? Will my marriage last?

It's impossible to live without fear—the best we can do is find the courage to work with the fears as they come up. Some of us deal with fear by asking, "What's the worst thing that could happen? Could I survive it?" Others take a more inward approach by asking, "Why am I afraid?" Both are good steps toward acknowledging that the fear is real and does need to be processed.

Lynn found a workable solution. "I decided one day that I could only deal with the fears I had that day. I found myself projecting so many of my thoughts into the future—especially regarding my children. I was tired of feeling afraid, so I decided to use a self-talk technique whenever a fear came up: I'd tell myself, 'Let that fear go. It hasn't happened, and if it does happen, you will deal with it then.' The more I'm able to let go of my future fears and deal with the fear I'm experiencing in that moment, the more competent I'm becoming at feeling the fear and facing it."

I learn what it means to be courageous each time I face my fear.

11.

Mom's Appointment Book

The quickest way for a parent to get a child's attention is to sit down and look comfortable.

—LANE OLINHOUSE

Years ago, when my children were still very young, I found a letter on my computer written by one of my babysitters. The letter was addressed to her mother and said, "What kind of mom has to make appointments with her own children? . . . I'll never make my kids feel like they are penciled into my schedule—who does she think she is?"

As I read, guilt overcame me, followed by anger. After a few minutes of rage, unsure whether to delete the letter, confront the babysitter, or pretend I'd never seen it, I started really thinking about my reasons for making appointments with my kids.

I had four children by the time I was thirty, and they were one to two years apart.

I set the appointments, not because my kids were penciled into my life, but because I wanted each of them to know how special they were to me. It wasn't the only time I saw my children, I reminded myself—but it was the only time I saw them individually.

During our appointed time I let each child decide exactly what we would do. My daughter did the same thing each week—we'd go to the park, and she'd sit in the tire swing and spin round and round while we sang songs and I watched dizzily. My son chose something that had to do with getting food—an ice cream cone, a candy bar from the store, a trip to the deli for a sandwich. I still remember these dates very clearly—exactly what we did, what we talked about, how I felt. They remember too—I asked my daughter this morning, and she told me all about the swing at the park.

We all organize our lives differently. It's hard to pay individual attention to a child when the commotion of family life is swirling round and round. Scheduled events, personal appointments—all have to fit somehow into a twenty-four-hour day. Finding time to spend one-on-one with your children creates lasting, loving memories, even if you have to pencil their names into your appointment book.

Having and keeping a schedule allows me to spend my time wisely.

12.

Everyday Magic

Luck is the residue of design,

— BRANCH RICKEY

I often use the words "good luck" in my everyday life. I sign letters with those words when I'm writing to someone who is facing some sort of challenge, I say them to my children before a game or a test, I even chant them silently over a manuscript before putting it in the mail. In all of these cases, the success or good fortune happens by chance *after* months of training, hard work, and preparation.

Luck, magic, the idea of something going on in the world that is unknown, fantastic, and beyond our control is a big part of the traditions of childhood, something many of us leave behind in our adult lives. We wish for good things to happen by chance so we can find fortune in our lives—but we forget about the everyday magic.

So I ask myself, where is the magic that has been sprinkled through my days? There is magic in every nook and cranny of my life—in the laughter at dinnertime, in the tulips that peak through the snow, in a surprise trip to the theater. Have I taken the time to collect these small nuggets of gold?

Once a friend gave me a small lucky pebble to hold in my hand when I had to face a difficult situation. She held it in her hand before giving it to me, talking to it, wishing to transfer the energy of luck into that small pebble to accompany me into this difficulty. I put it in my pocket and held on to it during the event—and I actually felt the energy she had put into that rock. It was in that moment that I figured out the truth about luck: the magic is in our minds. It is in our ability to imagine, to visualize, to create, and mostly to see our lives as lucky or unlucky. It's also in the faith of a good friend. That rock in my pocket was powerless without my belief that by chance what I wished (and worked for) would indeed happen. The pots of gold are invisible unless we choose to see them.

I choose to see and experience the magic in my life.

13.

A Giving Nature

Our deeds determine us, as much as we determine our deeds.

—GEORGE ELIOT

I had the honor of presenting a talk to families with children under five years old. The subject of the discussion was how to promote positive values and raise community-connected kids. One woman asked: "It is easy to get caught up in the daily activities of child-rearing, letting the goal of raising children with values fall to the back burner. How can we promote our children's giving natures?"

She wanted her five-year-old to think of others instead of being so focused on himself, and she wanted concrete ways to teach and support these valued life skills. All of us want to raise social-minded, compassionate children who are able to make a positive contribution to their school, family, and ultimately society as they grow and learn.

How we do this is woven into the fabric of our lives. Let's look at the daily activities of child-rearing: packing lunches, doing dishes, washing clothes, cleaning the house, playing with kids, preparing meals, planning activities, driving to friends' houses, bathing, hugging, and listening—just to name a few. We can say all we want about what we value. What we actually do, however, is what our children will imitate. You teach what you value with every action you take.

Sure there are things you can do to raise a child's or your family's awareness of others, like making donations to a food pantry, offering help to an older woman at the grocery store, or bringing food to a sick neighbor. But don't shortchange the significance of the everyday care you give. What is important to you becomes important to your children. How can we promote our children's giving natures? By being giving people ourselves—and then by praising every small effort we see as they learn to model all the behaviors we hope to teach.

I teach my children what I value with every action I take.

14.

The Welcome Mat

God does not ask your ability or your inability. He asks only your availability.

—MARY KAY ASH

Most Saturday nights our house is the place to be. That's because one of my goals has always been to make our home a place where everyone feels welcome. The plan obviously worked—just last weekend I counted thirteen kids sprawled across couches, on the floor, in my kids' rooms, and sleeping out on the trampoline.

When parents walk through our door on Sunday morning to pick up their kids, the house looks like a bomb went off—but I've learned to smile graciously, even if I'm still in my pajamas, and say, "The kids had a great time!" I no longer care what they think about the mess or the fact that so many kids are here. My kids are happy, their kids are happy—isn't that the goal?

Most of us want to establish the feeling of community in our lives. We want to have friends to celebrate with, to be invited to attend events, and to feel a connection with family and friends. We want our children to have many people they can turn to— people they know and like. This cannot be accomplished unless we are willing to open our homes to others.

The problem is that most of us have so many expectations that go along with any kind of entertaining. We don't think our home is presentable—we're waiting until we remodel the kitchen or put some grass on the pile of dirt that is our yard. Some of us believe that to invite friends to tea means we'd have to clean the bathrooms and bake cookies—which all takes too much time and energy.

We can find much happiness in the company of others if we just open our doors no matter what the circumstances, lower our expectations as to what kind of food or entertainment we'll need to provide, and simply offer welcoming arms.

Today I will put out the welcome mat and
build my personal community.

15.

We All Have Disabilities

I seldom think about my limitations, and they never make me sad. Perhaps there is just a touch of yearning at times; but it is vague, like a breeze among flowers.

—HELEN KELLER

There I stood in the middle of the cereal aisle with my five-year-old son lying flat on the floor, screaming, "You're mean," in his hard-to-understand English, louder than an alarm. I spoke in a tense, quiet voice into his ear: "Get up now. I mean it—you stop yelling." He yelled louder.

An older woman was trying to get around us with her cart, so I slid his body to one side of the aisle as I gave her an apologetic smile. She looked away as if I beat my son regularly. He had fits like this daily. Once I even thought of having a shirt printed for him to wear that would say, "I'm autistic. Life is too stimulating, so I scream sometimes—it's not my mother's fault."

Being a mother is hard enough without difficulties you didn't bargain for. Yet there is a secret that all mothers share: we will embrace and love whatever child comes into our lives.

Someone once told me that we all have disabilities—some are just more pronounced than others and present greater opportunities for growth. We take the first step toward acceptance by researching until we understand the disability, the drugs used, and the treatments possible. We then embark on the journey, enthusiastic and strong. But we also grieve along the way for the child we had hoped for and we cry over what our baby won't be able to do, be, or feel in this life.

Of course, along with the successes and lessons this very special child teaches us there are moments of defeat—when the other children make fun, or when your child cries out, "Why me? Why can't I be like everyone else?"

There is no answer to this question. No matter how many motivational stories you tell, the truth is that for this child life is going to be a struggle. But speaking as the mother of a child with disabilities, I can say that we *all* receive gifts beyond measure—we learn what it means to truly love unconditionally and we come to understand that strength of character can be learned.

I have the strength to embrace and love my children no matter what difficulty they present.

Nobody's Perfect— Including Mothers

If you have made mistakes . . . there is always another chance for you. . . . You may have a fresh start any moment you choose, for this thing we call "failure" is not the falling down, but the staying down.

—MARY PICKFORD

"Last week I was kind enough to do a load of laundry for my daughter," said Kate. "Unfortunately, I didn't look through the pile to see that two of the tops were dry-clean only. Well, they could have fit a doll by the time they were dried.

"My daughter was in tears—so angry at me for being careless. Of course, I had to mention that she was the one who put the clothes in the regular laundry basket—but that didn't seem to help. So I took this opportunity to remind her that mothers are allowed to make mistakes too!"

As mothers, we get many chances to make mistakes, but we don't usually point them out to our kids. In fact, often we defend ourselves, wanting to keep them thinking we are perfect in every way.

In reality, it is really important for our kids to see us making mistakes, feeling embarrassed, not succeeding at something, or admitting to an action we regret later. Kids do these things all the time and usually get caught in the act *and* corrected. So if we can rise above our own frustration and be willing to go out of our way to point out our mistakes, a huge lesson can be learned.

It's even better if you can point out the times you fail, the jobs you don't get, the papers you write that are rejected, and the friends who don't call you back. Kids learn how to handle the feelings that life brings simply by observing how you handle similar situations. A kid who hears his mother say, "I made a mistake," or, "I'm feeling sad that I didn't get this job," is going to know what to do when he breaks your favorite vase or doesn't make a sports team.

He'll know it is okay not to be perfect, that everyone makes mistakes, and, most important, that he's still loved.

My kids need to see me making mistakes—they learn a lot from how I deal with sadness, frustration, and failure.

17.

Learn to Disappoint Others

Nine-tenths of our suffering is caused by others not thinking so much of us as we think they ought.

—MARY LYON

A girlfriend in college loved to say, 'You can't please all the people all the time,'" said Jean. "I used to think that was just her way of getting out of sticky situations. Whenever an opportunity came up, like tickets to a concert, even when she had already made other plans, she would go with the event that sounded like more fun. Someone would end up hurt or mad, but she didn't really care. She had this easygoing belief that someone might be disappointed but it certainly wasn't going to be her.

"I, on the other hand, always seem to care too much about disappointing others. Many times I've done something I didn't want to do because I was afraid I might disappoint someone. When I was younger, it affected my choice of lovers. Now it determines the way I relate to my husband, employer, and friends, and it dictates what volunteer opportunities I agree to do."

Learning to disappoint others is no easy task for mothers who have spent years of their lives trying to please people—and that includes most of us! We are supermothers, able to leap tall homework assignments and swing from sewing thread! Yet many of us feel imprisoned by others' expectations, to the point of making decisions based on not wanting to let someone down.

Learning to disappoint others is what I call a freedom skill. Once you learn to do it, you are forever free to make choices that please you—choices that may take others into consideration but not always put them first. Acceptance of the fact that you are going to disappoint people regularly, maybe even every day, allows you some space to breathe, move, and experiment with your life.

Today, instead of carefully placing my foot on life's path, I will walk boldly even if I disappoint someone in the process.

18.

Ten Minutes a Day

The most beautiful thing we can experience is the mysterious. It is the source of all true art and all science. He to whom this emotion is a stranger, who can no longer pause to wonder and stand rapt in awe, is as good as dead: his eyes are closed.

—ALBERT EINSTEIN

I took the weekend off, left my kids with my mom and dad, and headed up to Ashland, Oregon, with my husband," said Darla, the mother of three. "What is most profound for me on these couples' getaways (aside from not cooking, sleeping in, and getting to do whatever I want) is the silence. There are no video games playing or overloaded washing machines bouncing around. Instead, I sit with windows open, listening to birds and watching leaves blow softly in the breeze. In this space, I can hear my own voice. There is room to dream."

As mothers, we have an ability to organize our thoughts on many tracks. Track one might be the things we have to do that day: pick up kids and groceries, see about school projects that are due, pay bills—the usual things. On track two might be a specific problem one of the kids is having. Track three might be a relationship issue or perhaps a friend who is sick. These many tracks pull our emotions in a daily tug-of-war as we try our best to manage it all. We have so many tracks to attend to that we seldom develop a track devoted to ourselves.

This is where sitting in silence comes in. If we can turn down the volume of our lives for even ten minutes a day, we might be able to hear ourselves. This quiet time does not have to be in a secluded room lit with candles or deep in a beautiful forest. Silence can be found in everyday moments.

When you're driving the car alone, turn off the radio. When you sip a cup of tea, do it outside on your porch without a paper, magazine, or list in your hand. Make an effort to listen to your thoughts instead of figuring out the next few hours, days, or months of your life. Don't lose yourself in the noise—instead, choose to create space for yourself within the silence.

I will create a space for silence in my everyday moments.

19.

An Inspiring Habit

Our strength is often composed of the weakness we're damned if we're going to show.

—MIGNON MCLAUGHLIN

I was at my neighbor Sue's house the other day and noticed a quote taped to her refrigerator. When I used the bathroom, I saw a quote taped on the mirror above the sink as well. Upon returning to finish my cup of tea, I asked her about her "quote" habit.

It had begun two years before when her mother died. Friends had sent letters of condolence with wonderful thoughts about her mother that she wanted to remember, so she wrote them up on index cards and hung them up at various locations around the house. Sue said that the notes made the process of grieving much easier. "It was like being surrounded by all the people who loved and missed my mom as much as I did," she said.

A few months later Sue decided she needed a new batch of inspiration on the topic of friendship. Her mother had been her best friend, and Sue felt it was time she met some new people. But she was a shy person who needed constant encouragement and reminders of the benefits of friendship to gain the courage to step out of her house and make the effort.

There are many times in our lives when we don't feel quite ready to face the world, and we need a little nudging to make us believe we can live the kind of life we want to live. Often we know what trait we are missing, or where confidence is lacking. Like Sue, we could all benefit by surrounding ourselves with thoughts that inspire us to keep moving in a positive, life-affirming direction.

Perhaps we can pick a thought for each day, carry it around with us, and use it to replace any negative, doubtful, or fear-producing thought. Maybe we want to tape the thoughts up in an inconspicuous place, where only we will hear the gentle nudging. Or maybe we put them up in clear view, sharing them with friends and family. Our lives are created minute by minute by the thoughts we have. So we need to surround ourselves with words, ideas, and thoughts that nurture our spirits.

The way I think determines the way I live.

What It Really Means to Have Style

Let the world know you as you are, not as you think you should be, because sooner or later, if you are posing, you will forget the pose, and then where are you?

—FANNIE BRICE

It was in the eighth grade when I first understood what it meant to have style," said Molly, the mother of three young girls. "I was telling my mother how much I wished I could look like a girl in my class. My mother said, 'You are ten times more beautiful than she is—she just has style. She knows how to put clothes together, fix her hair, and act in a way that makes her stand out.'

"My mother helped shift my perception of beauty that day," Molly continued. "From then on, all I wanted was to somehow obtain my own style."

Often we focus too much attention on whether we possess the current definition of beauty. We critique our facial features and complain, "I'd be pretty if not for my nose (small lips, lack of eyelids, large thighs)!"

The face and body we're born with is out of our control; we have what we have. But style—that's another matter altogether.

Style can evolve, shift, or be reinvented whenever you like. It is your unique way of expressing the woman you are at any given point in your life.

So how do we obtain this style? How, with limited time and resources, do we suddenly achieve this put-together, uniquely ourselves look? It begins with a desire to express ourselves, followed by the courage to step off the treadmill of other people's definitions of beauty. It also takes some thought—if you haven't spent much time focused on your personal style, you may have no idea what you want that style to be.

Look around—start noticing the clothes that make you feel good when you wear them. Try doing your hair a different way or stop by a makeup counter for a free makeover. Experiment! Have the courage to try out different looks, and actually leave your house in them. Don't be afraid to be an original.

Discovering my personal style is a fun
and creative way to express myself.

21.

Actions Speak Louder

It is easier to act your way into new ways of feeling than to feel yourself into new ways of acting.

—SUSAN GLASER

When my children reached the age when they started to argue with me (somewhere around four!), I began a ritual I learned from my college roommate. After living together in the same apartment for a few months, Bonnie and I had a small argument. I remember waking up around midnight to see her sitting on my bed. She said quietly, "We really shouldn't close our eyes to sleep with a problem left between us."

Her small act of love, thoughtfulness, and respect toward our growing friendship made its mark, and I've remembered it ever since. I began doing the same thing with my children when they were young, in small ways that seemed insignificant. But as they grew older those trips to their bedrooms at night weren't as easy. Often I'd be the one apologizing, having to admit I'd lost my temper or didn't listen well enough.

The other night my sixteen-year-old daughter, Brooke, and I were having a discussion about the car she wanted to buy. She is buying this car herself, so really the choice is hers and depends on how much money she can come up with. But for some reason we began arguing. I thought she should look at something less expensive and not so "cool." She said that she had worked for the summer so she could buy something she really wanted. The conversation ended abruptly. About ten o'clock the telephone rang. It was Brooke: "Mom, I guess I've become like you. I can't go to sleep. I feel bad about the way our conversation ended."

My theory on mothering is constantly affirmed—children learn *everything* by watching what we *do*. What we say has little impact if it isn't backed up by personal action. So as hard as it seems sometimes, be true to who you are, and you'll raise kids who will do the same!

What I do today matters.

22.

Too Stressed for Sex

I discovered I always have choices and sometimes it's only a choice of attitude.

—JUDITH M. KNOWLTON

I know I'm not the only mom who is too tired to make love," said Linda. "Around lunchtime the idea sounds doable. I still feel relaxed, rested, and can fantasize about being touched. But come 9:00 p.m., after putting my kids to bed, rubbing backs, telling stories, and doing dishes, I've had as much stimulus as I can handle. My husband reaches out to touch me, and I have to tell him apologetically that I can't handle one more person needing me. I actually feel sorry for him, but I feel sorry for me too—I can't figure out what happened to that wild woman who couldn't wait to rip his clothes off.

"Sometimes we even discuss ways to make my evenings less stressful so I'll feel like making love—usually that involves my leaving the house entirely. I've gotten to the stage where even a PTA meeting can produce sexual thoughts simply by removing me from the emotional energy in the house for an hour! My husband has volunteered to do all the homework, take care of the dishes, even cook the dinner, if the end result is that I am relaxed enough to make love."

Many of us feel like Linda. We might be too tired, or maybe we've lost interest in sex with everything else that's going on in our lives. Whatever the reason, guilt is usually part of the equation—we know our man wants it, and we wish we wanted it, but we don't. Perhaps it is time to be more realistic and to accept the fact that mothering is a tough job that might indeed lower a woman's sex drive. Part of loving ourselves includes gaining knowledge and acceptance of our true feelings, even when those feelings aren't exactly what we want them to be. Unless we are honest with ourselves about how we do feel, it is impossible to change or improve things.

There may be practical ways to help us feel more amorous, like a massage, weekends away, a dinner we haven't cooked, or an evening out with a friend. But in the meantime, during the lull and before the next hormonal spurt that puts sex back on your radar screen, embrace the woman you are right now.

I am a beautiful, sensual, and engaging woman
even when I don't feel like making love.

23.

Let Go of the Rope

A woman is like a teabag—you can't tell how strong she
is until you put her in hot water.

—NANCY REAGAN

As mothers we must constantly assert ourselves, because
our children are constantly asserting themselves," said
Meg, a single mother of two adolescent girls. "In a way it is a war
of wills. Sometimes I find myself backing down, feeling sorry
after I give a consequence for a bad behavior, not wanting my
kids to miss some fun event. When I come home late at night to
find the sink full of dishes, even though I know I should go wake
up the responsible person, I find myself doing the dishes instead.

"I often struggle to assert myself with my daughter, who is
decidedly stronger-willed than me. Am I just too nice? Do I compromise before I need to? If I visualize a tug-of-war, with me on
one side and the kids on the other, I realize that the only way to
win is to let go of the rope, to stop pulling and start asking what
it is I really want them to learn from me. When they are sitting
on the ground with the slack rope in their hands, then I can
explain that it isn't really the sink full of dishes that bothers me;
it is the lack of thoughtfulness. It isn't coming in late that is the
problem; it is the lying about it."

Children need boundaries; they crave the security that limits
offer—they want us to stand by the rules and expectations we

set, even when they fight with us to change them. Every time we feel pushed or pulled, manipulated or lied to, we must remember that old saying, "The buck stops here." Whether we want to be the heavy or not, the job is ours.

We must allow our own spirit to constantly assert itself; the part of us that loves, creates, plans, nurtures, and believes in justice has to shine forth. We need to show up fully aware of our power as women and as mothers and trust ourselves to rule fairly and rightly.

Today I will be the assertive one.

24.

The Real Think Tank

You have to leave the city of your comfort and go into the wilderness of your intuition. What you'll discover will be wonderful. What you'll discover will be yourself.

—ALAN ALDA

I usually smile as I listen to women talking with each other— it's like witnessing a think tank in progress. One behavior women learn from an early age is to ask each other's opinions. We want to get a consensus that what we are considering is the right thing, so often we wait until the people most important to us have given us their vote—and then we move forward.

This allows us to think out loud as we talk to each person about the decision confronting us. It proves that we have an open mind and are willing to hear different viewpoints, and it gives us the time we need to process what is going on.

The only problem with this way of making a decision is that we can forget how we really feel—or worse, we may not even ask ourselves what we want or think before we head out to gather the opinions of others. It is almost as if other people's ideas or direction for us would offer better solutions than what we can find within our own hearts.

My friend Amanda had to make a decision about where she would send her son to school the next year. She said she'd made a list of the good and bad points but had gone over it so many times that she was stuck—she didn't know what was best anymore.

I believed that she absolutely knew what the right choice was, so we tried an experiment. I asked her to sit quietly, take a few deep breaths, and then, with a clear mind, ask herself what school was best for David. Next, she was to write down the very first answer that popped into her mind. Within less than five minutes Amanda looked at the answer on her paper with a big smile on her face.

Mothers have an amazing capacity to *know*—it's called intuition. We know the answer to most of the questions, dilemmas, and problems we face. All we need to do is quiet the many voices around us, center ourselves, and be willing to listen. Sometimes our intuition is the only think tank we need.

Before I ask others for direction, I will ask myself and write it down. That way I won't get lost along the way.

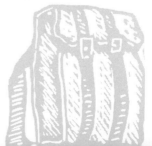

Both Right and Wrong

Where there is great love, there are always miracles.

—WILLA CATHER

It was an exciting day when my seventeen-year-old made her first big decision as an adult. I decided to leave the college application process up to her, explaining that I'd be there to answer questions, read over essays, or help in whatever way I could, but that ultimately choosing a college, applying, and being accepted would be her job. Then I sat back and watched.

So many times during the past seventeen years I'd doubted my choices, worried about whether my parenting approach was working, whether the latest book on discipline was right, or whether I was teaching my daughter the life skills she would need to survive in the world. I made mistakes. She experienced one traumatic event after another—divorce, moving from house to house, changing schools, struggling with an abusive coach and the blending of a new family. My parenting style fluctuated according to the struggles in my own life—sometimes I was exceptional, but at other times I was depressed and overwhelmed.

I realized as I proudly watched her accept a sports scholarship to the university of her choice, after doing all the work to contact the coach herself, that nothing I did right or wrong created the daughter I saw standing in front of me.

Because I did both right and wrong. The only consistent ingredient in her life has been my love for her and my belief in her right to determine the girl, and now woman, that she wants to be. There were many times I cried as I watched her struggle or face the consequences of her actions. I tried my best not to jump in to save her—sometimes I was successful; other times I wasn't.

Unconditional love is the most valuable gift we give to our children. Everything else flows from that—our support, the ability to forgive, and the belief that our children can do anything they dream of. So forget the parenting instruction manuals. Instead, look to your own inner voice—your loving voice—for instruction and guidance.

I love my children enough to let them grow into
the people they are meant to be.

26.

Seize the Moment

The strongest principle of growth lies in human choice.

—GEORGE ELIOT

Late on Sunday night I returned from a movie to find my car packed with skis, a snowboard, boots, and chains for the tires. On the kitchen counter was a note: "Mom, Rhett and I decided to go skiing in the morning—why don't you come with us? We're leaving at 5:30."

First you have to know that I'm *not* a morning person. Even the usual time of 6:45 finds me stumbling around the kitchen trying to remember who likes what in their lunch. So the idea of getting up, driving three hours to ski, and then trying to keep up with the kids all day on the slopes was not that appealing.

As mothers go, I'm as flexible as the next—a change in plans is par for the course. But this was going to put a lot of pressure on the rest of my week. So at first I told myself that they would have more fun without me, that a little brother-sister bonding would be good for them. And then I started thinking that next year at this time my daughter would be in college far away from me. How many other opportunities would I have to spend a carefree day riding up ski lifts and chatting?

I knew I'd made the right decision when we pulled out of the driveway in the still dark morning and the CD that blasted from the speakers was Elton John's greatest hits, which is not my children's favorite. Rhett then said, "I put in Elton John for you because I know you like him."

On this day I set my reasoning aside and listened to my heart. As a result, I was reminded of how important it is to create a little extra space in our lives so that if our responsibilities have to be set aside for an hour, a day, or a week, we won't be thrown into a state of panic. We have to seize the moments that are offered to us, because often the opportunity doesn't come again.

I will discover new ways to play with my children this week!

A Life of Spiritual Practice

We must overcome the notion that we must be regular. . . .
It robs you of the chance to be extraordinary and leads
you to the mediocre.

—UTA HAGEN

Years ago I was lucky to stumble onto a program that offered spiritual direction. I wasn't sure exactly what it was, but I figured that I could use direction—spiritual or otherwise—so I signed up. At the first meeting I told my director how difficult it was for me to adhere to any regular spiritual practice, whether it be praying, doing yoga, or sitting in the garden to meditate. I would make a plan, schedule the time, do the practice for a few days, and quit.

She asked what I thought were kind of silly questions about making dinner, time spent with my children, housekeeping, my work, and all the other little things I do each day. As I answered and listened, it dawned on me that she was trying to say that my life *was* my spiritual practice. She said that monks and other religious people may have time to meditate, to pray, and to live lives of solitude dedicated to their spiritual practices, but I was living a much more difficult existence. Imagine that—my life, simply in living it, was teaching me what the mystics sitting in their caves were trying to learn.

"Yes," she said. "You have opportunities every hour to pay attention to your thoughts, even while you're making dinner. You love, sacrifice, and set your own needs aside many times each day—that is what spirit seekers are trying to learn. What is prayer really, and what is a spiritual practice?"

I didn't know the answer, but I understood and embraced her belief that my life could be my prayer if I devoted my whole heart to it. That insight changed the way I lived each day. The mundane, usual jobs became my spiritual practice. I didn't need to be sitting in meditation to learn to focus my mind—I had kids to listen to. I'd weed the garden, dig my hands into the dirt, and express my gratitude in the connection I felt to the earth.

When I'm tempted to look outside myself to find the self-improvement I think I need, I will remember to pay attention to what I already do and have. This can be the answer I seek

28.

Creative? Yes—You!

The creative act, the defeat of habit by originality, overcomes everything.

—GEORGE LOIS

Not long ago a friend stopped by while I was working on a tile mosaic for my kitchen wall. She rubbed her fingers over the bright birds that were taking shape and sighed, "I wish I were creative like you." I handed her the tray of tiles and a bowl of glue and told her to help me while she listened to the lecture I planned to deliver.

"Women are blessed with a creative soul," I began. "It is naturally in us. Sometimes we haven't found opportunities in our lives to experience the extent of our creative power—but that doesn't mean the ability isn't there." I went on to point out her three children—"What is more creative than giving birth to a human being?" I asked. She nodded her head but didn't look too convinced.

"Each day we use our imagination to make decisions—we create meals, choose our clothing, decorate our homes, plan our family events—all of these activities offer opportunities to expand our creative process. A mother's life is the epitome of the creation cycle. As our children enter each new stage, we seek knowledge, we modify our parenting approach, and we engage in all sorts of activities that expand our thoughts as well as our children's talents. See how many ways you create?" I said, ending my monologue.

Our lives can feel out of focus at times—our children have events we need to get them to, homework that has to be done, and everyone has to be fed, clothed, and nurtured. It is in turning to our creative nature, within the everyday structure of our lives, that we find the courage to grow into the woman we want to be. Maybe it's been a while since you've picked up a paintbrush or danced alone in your kitchen. Perhaps you stopped singing long ago, have forgotten about your favorite book of poetry, or stored away your photography equipment when the baby was born. It is never too late to tap into the powerful stream of creative juices inside of you—to find it and then marvel at its ability to heal you.

> *I claim my right to use my imagination—*
> *to be original and to engage in a creative activity just*
> *for the fun of it, with no goal in mind.*

29.

The Men in Your Life

Insanity: doing the same thing over and over again and expecting different results.

—ALBERT EINSTEIN

As I sign my dad's Father's Day card I'm reminded of how important it is to have men in our lives whom we can count on. When I look back over the past ten years, my father's face has almost always been in the crowd of supporters. Whether it's one of my kids' sporting events, a talk I'm giving at a local bookstore, or financial support for summer camps—he's there ready to back me up.

I have brothers too—who know how to listen, who offer great advice, who model the kind of life values I want my children to emulate. My husband has enthusiastically and lovingly taken on the lives, issues, joys, successes, and everyday struggles of four children who aren't his by birth. The list goes on—men who stepped into my life while I was going through my divorce—teachers, coaches, friends' fathers, neighbors.

I talked with a girlfriend yesterday and asked her what it was about her husband that made their relationship so great. She said that twenty years ago, when they first married, he supported her as she struggled with the transition into motherhood. He replaced each thought of self-doubt with an affirmation of her abilities, gifts, and talents. He held her up both emotionally and physically, never taking his sights off the importance of her health in supporting the family he loved.

If this kind of support sounds foreign to you, it may be a good time to ask yourself why. Hundreds of books have been written on the differences between men and women, and they tell us that there are behaviors we need to accept because it is "just how men are." I don't believe this anymore. The older I get and the more women I talk with, the more obvious the truth becomes—men treat us how we allow them to treat us.

We want men in our lives as lovers, friends, and supporters. Our children need them as role models, fathers, teachers, and partners. It's important to step back and look at the men in your life and ask some important questions: How do you allow them to treat you? Do you have the kind of relationships you really want?

I will surround myself and my children with men
who treat us with love and respect.

Show Up as Yourself

Intimacy is being seen and known as the person you truly are.

—AMY BLOOM

I t's true that making love creates more intimacy in a relation-ship, but it is also true that lack of an intimate connection within the everyday moments makes sex impossible. We all know what it feels like to have intimacy—or not. When we sense this connection, everything in our relationship feels great; we look forward to our time spent together, can't wait to get our partner on the phone to ask an opinion, and are open in our lovemaking.

When we start to feel resentful, taken for granted, unloved, or rejected, we retreat into ourselves, unable to open up to what-ever intimacy might be offered. What once was a love relation-ship starts to feel more like being roommates. The distressing thing about this cycle is that men think they can create intimacy with sex, so they push in that direction, while women need the intimacy in everyday ways in order to feel like having sex. Nobody gets what he or she wants or needs, so lovers grow fur-ther apart.

Yet if you understand how the cycle of intimacy works, it isn't that hard to create. All you need is the courage to show up in the relationship as yourself—with the skill to say exactly what you think, feel, dream, and fear. If your partner has the ability to really listen *and* hear you without judgment, projection of personal expectations, or the need to be right, you have all you will ever need to be intimate partners. Of course, both of you need to possess and use these skills at all times! That's the hard part. The truth, however, is that it takes far less time to learn and use these skills than it does to heal the relationship once you've drifted apart.

I will find fifteen minutes today to really listen to my partner, then find it again tomorrow and the next day. The energy will shift, intimacy will grow, and both of us will find that we have exactly what we need and want.

31.

Bathing Suit Blues

There is a fountain of youth: it is your mind, your talents, the creativity you bring to your life and the lives of people you love. When you learn to tap this source, you will have truly defeated age.

—SOPHIA LOREN

Vacation is approaching—that dreaded time of year when I'll have to consider wearing a bathing suit. I sit and page through old family photo albums and wonder: Whatever happened to the bathing suits that looked more like tennis dresses?

The ones that covered an inch or so of your inner thigh? The kind that didn't require shaving your bikini line daily?

I often wonder why they don't sell bathing suits according to age instead of size. It isn't right that my sixteen-year-old and I are thumbing through the same racks. Oh, I don't want to make it sound like there are no options for the older woman—there are the suits with cups that could double as bulletproof vests.

But it is more than the suit itself that bothers me—it is the concept. What makes us think we're supposed to look good in a bathing suit at forty years old? Have we missed some step in our development having to do with accepting reality? Skin does sag no matter how many Pilates classes we attend. Shouldn't there be a time in our lives when we can stop worrying about the shape of our bodies?

Of course, we each have the option of accepting ourselves whatever size we are—and some of us acquire the wisdom to step out of the "beauty at all costs" (including major surgery) game. But what happens if you're stuck somewhere in between—sometimes wanting to look fit, thin, and young, and at other times determined to give yourself the break you've earned?

How do we really come to terms with the aging process? Well, we could start by watching the way men approach aging: leave the gray hair, gain twenty pounds, give up running for card-playing, and drink more beer. But if we're serious about entering midlife in a healthy state of mind, we should start asking ourselves the questions that matter: What do I want? Can I be happy with the body I have instead of wanting something different? Is there a bathing suit designer out there who cares?

My body is a beautiful masterpiece.

32

Let Tears Rain

We need never be ashamed of our tears.

—CHARLES DICKENS

Spring is the season when the most rain falls. After the rain, plants grow at amazing speed; they bloom bright and full. When we allow our tears to fall, we grow too," said Amber. "Years ago when my kids were all in elementary school, a therapist I'd been seeing for depression asked me if I ever cried in front of my kids. I told her that I couldn't remember a time when my kids had seen me cry. When I was sad or upset, I went to my room, or I waited until I took a shower and cried when nobody could hear me.

"The therapist then told me that my assignment that week was to cry in front of my kids and see what happened. I questioned this assignment. It would ruin everything I'd worked so hard to build—I'd done everything to make sure my kids saw me as a happy mother. She then told me that I was robbing my children of a real life skill they needed to be comfortable with—crying. By acting as if I was having a great day when in fact something had happened that upset me, I was teaching them to stuff and hide their feelings just as I was.

"It took a few days. I argued with my husband early that morning but pulled myself together to get the kids up and ready for school. When my husband left for work, he walked out the door without saying good-bye. I tried to hold back the tears but then remembered that I was supposed to cry. My daughter noticed my tears and came over to give me a hug, asking what was wrong. I told her I was feeling very sad because her father and I had an argument and he hadn't said good-bye.

"It was so simple, so healing, and it changed the way I interacted with my kids. All of a sudden I didn't have to be this fountain of enthusiasm and joy every minute of the day. I could be real. I learned how to embrace my tears, and with that came the ability to define, recognize, and honor my feelings."

Tears are like rain—necessary for cleansing and growth.

33.

Controlled Burn

It is not the strongest of the species that survive, not the most intelligent, but the one most responsive to change.

—CHARLES DARWIN

W hen I was young, I used to watch the firemen tending the controlled-burn areas around our town," said Jill. "The concept intrigued me—to burn something in advance so it wouldn't be the cause of a greater fire. When I turned thirty-five, I did a controlled burn of my own! I made a long list of all the catalysts for fires in my life: the negative thoughts I had, friends who continually brought me down, organizations I'd volunteered for that I no longer enjoyed, and activities that no longer fed my soul.

"One particular responsibility sticks out in my mind. I'd been president of a women's club for a long time—three or four years. I felt overwhelmed, unable to enjoy my service any longer.

"I didn't need firemen. All I needed was more courage than I'd had in the past and a few days with a telephone in my hand. I called each of the members on the board of our women's club and told them I resigned. As I checked off the items on my burn list, I became lighter and lighter—to the point of euphoria."

Many of us feel that life is bringing us down, but we aren't sure why. We haven't looked ahead and decided which areas of our life to burn so that we aren't fighting bigger fires, ones that occupy all of our time and energy. We think we are stuck with our friends, our volunteer activities, and our jobs even if we feel they are sucking the life out of us. Yet if we are brave enough to investigate all areas of our lives, looking for the people, activities, or experiences that continually bring us down, and are willing to do something about removing them, we are able to make room for things that fill us with new energy.

This feeling of freedom may feel very strange at first. You may even feel selfish for putting your needs first—but the doubt will pass, and in no time you'll feel renewed and alive.

I will think "controlled burn"—and get started on my list.

34

Fire the Judge

It is hard to fight an enemy who has outposts in your head.

—SALLY KEMPTON

I have this judge who lives in my head," said Karen, the mother of two teenage boys. "My judge sits on a big purple sofa, in her flowered house dress, drinking lemonade as she points her finger at me. I hear her voice when I'm opening the refrigerator to get a snack, deciding whether or not to take a vacation, or finding the courage to wear sexy lingerie. In general my judge never says an encouraging thing —instead, she points out all the ways I could be better, prettier, more lovable, or more accomplished.

"The really sad thing is that I actually listen to her and believe what I hear. Sometimes I negotiate with my judge: I try to convince her that one cupcake will not make me fat, or that I'm due for a little time off. She may even agree, but there's always a *but* in her sentence. 'Yes, you do need a break, *but* what about that project you promised to complete?' 'I can see you want that cupcake, *but* you won't fit into the dress you just bought.'

"I've been thinking about my judge a lot. I figure that if I'm letting her live rent-free in my head, at least I should get something out of it. I hired her, created her, have allowed her free rein—so I also have the power to fire her or change the job description!"

Most of us have a voice that lives in our head and gives an opinion or judgment about the way we choose to live our lives. For a moment imagine your judge—put a face and body to the voice. See a finger wagging at you, telling you what you should or shouldn't do. Then imagine the wagging finger turning into two hands applauding your choice. The next time the voice of judgment rings out in your mind, use your imagination and turn the judge into a figure you can laugh at—add angel's wings or giant's feet. You own this creature that lives in your head, so put it to work doing something that might inspire you!

There is no space for negative self-judgment in my life.

35.

Invitation to Your Defiant, Ass-kicking, Experimental Self

And the trouble is, if you don't risk anything, you risk even more.

—ERICA JONG

Remember sneaking out of the window to meet a friend, smoking in the garage, the secrets you kept, the friends you could count on, telling the truth no matter what anyone thought, dying your hair green, piercing a body part—the teen years?

Then we grew up and things began to matter; we were supposed to be responsible, had a reputation to uphold, and became role models for our own children. Still, somewhere inside the heart of that risk-taker still lives the girl who sought excitement in life over pleasing others, the girl who had less to lose.

What are the risks we turn away from as adults? What don't we do simply because we are afraid? Some of the hard choices we're faced with now include telling the truth, confronting someone, leaving a career we hate, loving someone we're afraid won't love us back, standing up for a cause, or confronting an abusive partner.

Remember the show *Let's Make a Deal?* The host would show contestants a TV or other prize and tell them that the prize was theirs or they could trade it for what was behind door number 1, door number 2, or door number 3. The catch was that one of the doors had nothing behind it. Would you settle for the TV or take a risk and see whether you could get something much better? How about when you were twenty—would it have been the TV or the unknown quantity behind the door?

The ability to take a risk depends on having the courage to experiment with life, to see what might happen if. . . . Fear of failure is what keeps us from climbing out of our current life window into the choices we only dream about. That's why we need to visit our teen souls and invite that fearless, defiant, ass-kicking, experimental, world-conquering part of us to come back and live alongside the thoughts that keep holding us back.

I am a woman who is willing and ready to take risks.

36

Listen to Your Anger

You need to claim the events of your life to make yourself yours. When you truly possess all you have been and done, which may take some time, you are fierce with reality.

—FLORIDA SCOTT MAXWELL

When I found out my husband was having an affair, I felt angry enough to strangle him," said Mandy, the mother of two preschoolers. "My therapist told me to embrace my anger, which made me laugh, since that would have meant spending the rest of my life in jail after killing him! After a few therapy sessions, I understood that what she really meant was to let my anger live, let it be okay with me, let it have a voice, and pay attention to what it was telling me."

Too many women make a habit of stuffing their anger—setting it aside for the good of the marriage, pretending its cause is PMS, or deciding before voicing it that nothing can be done so why bother. The problem is that the anger festers—it lives within us and builds on itself until we blow like a volcano at the slightest thing. Then we tell ourselves that we're unbalanced, depressed, moody, or bitchy—and apologize, or let it go, without finding out why we are angry.

What would it mean to let our anger live? It would mean that we welcome it into our feeling life with as much respect as we give to love, sadness, or any other emotion. Then we might sit with it for a few minutes—or an hour, or a day—pondering what it might be trying to teach us about a relationship, an experience, or ourselves.

Next we would respect the message we receive from our anger and be willing to do something about it. Doing something might mean setting clearer personal boundaries or even leaving a marriage or friendship—often the message implies an action of some sort. If you are angry with your spouse because you end up doing much more of the housework or dinner preparation, the action is to reassign household responsibilities. If you're angry at how a teacher has treated your child, the action is to make a phone call and talk about the incident.

What we don't want to do is pretend that our anger is a side effect of something else, a feeling to be embarrassed about or afraid of. Anger has a strong message, one that needs to be listened to and worked with, not cast aside as insignificant.

I respect my anger and allow it to teach me.

37.

Count to Ten
and Breathe!

Risk! Risk anything! Care no more for the opinion of others,
for those voices. Do the hardest thing on earth for you. Act
for yourself. Face the truth.

—KATHERINE MANSFIELD

When it comes to defending my children, sometimes it's hard to stand by the values I try to instill. Since school began, three boys have relentlessly taunted my learning-disabled son. The school is working on this problem, but I also know that middle school can be tough—and that kids get teased no matter what. I try to take it lightly and tell him to just ignore what is going on—until he comes home and reports something that puts me back on the warpath.

This past month has given me a better understanding of why violence is alive and well in our schools. Even I want revenge on these boys who have inflicted such pain on someone I love. Yesterday, while discussing what Troy might do, I told him not to push them or hit them at school, but if they were on our street after school, he could go ahead and hit them. My husband gasped, looked at me in shock, and proceeded to tell Troy that he could not hit them unless he was hit first. "But they deserve a consequence for their behavior," I fumed. All this from a woman who has banned TV, confiscated violent video games, and forbids music that promotes fighting!

Knowing and living what we believe in and value must determine our choice of actions even when the experience hits close to home. Given time to rethink my vengeful statement, I've decided to modify our bully plan and begin with negotiation (a phone call to the boys' parents).

I'm challenged to live by the values I believe in—that violence is never the answer and that peace and understanding are possible. As mothers, we experience our children's pain at a deep level, sometimes deeper than our children do. It hurts to watch them suffer, and yet it is what teaches us new coping strategies. It is the struggle that stretches our hearts and makes us stronger.

I know what I believe in and what I value.
My goal is to live by those standards

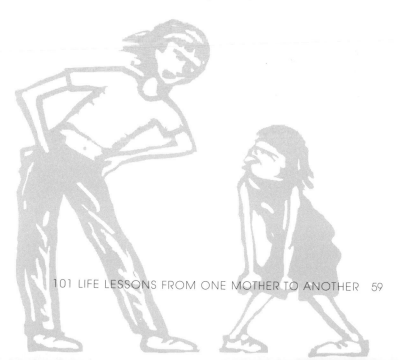

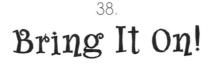

38.

Bring It On!

You gain strength, courage, and confidence by every experience in which you really stop to look fear in the face. . . . You must do the thing which you think you cannot do.

—ELEANOR ROOSEVELT

Over the last ten years I've done a lot of professional coaching on the subject of facing fears," said Grace, an inspirational speaker. "At home I find myself doing the same kind of coaching.

"Last weekend I watched my fourteen-year-old daughter warming up for an important basketball game against a better and more talented team. I marveled at her composure, confidence, and obvious excitement. Every movement in her body shouted: 'Bring it on!'

"Some people learn how to use fear to motivate them, to make them stronger, to give them the strength or desire to compete. My daughter has that gift. She may be afraid, but you'd never know it. I, on the other hand, have had to work very hard to overcome my fears. I still wake up in the middle of the night scared of an upcoming speech or worried about the next day's exhausting schedule."

We learn to be courageous by confronting and then working through our fears. That means we learn to feel the fear and move forward anyway. With each step, self-confidence grows.

As moms, we don't have as many opportunities to put our-selves out there, to try new things, to make choices that we might be afraid to make. Yet it is important to find those oppor-tunities and take a lesson from our kids who have benefited from the years of coaching that we ourselves have given them. We need to go for it, to not be afraid, and to believe that we can do whatever it is we set our heart and mind to!

I am a strong and courageous woman who is willing to try new things—and that includes learning from my children!

39.

Draw a Line in the Sand

Morality, like art, means drawing a line someplace.

—OSCAR WILDE

L ast week I had to make a difficult decision—whether or not to invite my kids' stepmother to a graduation party at my home," recounted Liza, the mother of three teenage boys. "First I decided to invite her since she plays an active role in my sons' lives. But then I knew I'd feel uncomfortable with her in my house. She had an affair with my husband, which precipitated the end of our marriage. Granted, that was ten years ago, and I know I should be over it by now, but I'm not.

"This is a big day for me," she continued. "My eldest son is graduating from high school. I'll probably be too busy to see her anyway. If I don't invite her, I'll feel guilty, but if I do, I'll resent it."

There are many opportunities in our lives to draw a line in the sand—to claim our right to set personal boundaries. Women often have a hard time drawing those lines. After a week of debating, Liza chose not to invite the stepmother.

It is easy to set boundaries when we don't care what others think of us. But most of us were raised to be people-pleasers. We find it hard to exclude someone, even if we know he or she has talked behind our backs. We let abusive people back into our homes. We try very hard not to make waves.

However, if we want to be powerful, effective, and truthful women, we need to learn to draw these lines. We need to be able to turn inward and believe that we have a right to set personal boundaries—even if others don't like the lines we've drawn!

I have a right to set boundaries based
solely on my desire to do so.

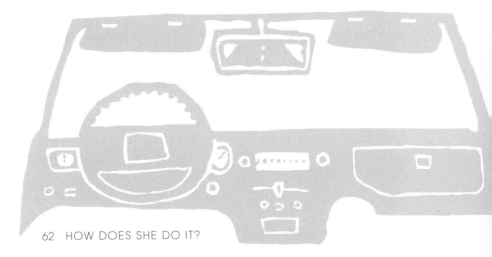

40.

Driving Lessons

It's frightening to think that you mark your children merely by being yourself. It seems unfair. You can't assume the responsibility for everything you do—or don't do.

—SIMONE DE BEAUVOIR

Every negative trait you ever possessed shows up when you're trying to teach a child to drive. A perfectly calm mother will scream at the top of her lungs as the child heads down a one-way street, oblivious to the suggestion of turning around. Threats abound—"If you don't do what I say the second I say it, I refuse to drive with you. You almost killed us!" The goal of building self-esteem is forgotten—"You absolutely may not drive with anyone but me in the car—until you're twenty-one!" A perfectly good relationship slips into blame and shame—"I saw you talking on the cell phone when you were driving with Dad. Don't you care at all about the people you might kill while driving so poorly?"

Of course, all of these interactions occur because we are afraid—for our children *and* our lives. This experience isn't so different from the feelings we had while teaching them to ride a bike, ski, be a good friend, or fall in love without breaking their heart. It's out of our control. We can tell them how, we can direct and show them, but in the end it will be their own bodies, minds, and decisions that will keep them safe—or not.

So we concentrate on our teacher's role, making sure they are the best they can be. We want to see that they are competent—actually more than competent. We don't want them to make any mistake, because a mistake could land them in the hospital, the principal's office, a police car, or the throes of a broken heart. On the one hand, we want our children to be courageous risk-takers who are sure of themselves—adults who feel competent. But on the other hand, we aren't sure if we are truly ready to give them the wheel of their own lives.

We go through this process whenever our children enter new stages, try new things, or choose sports (or other events) that scare us—tightening our grip when we feel something is slipping out of our control. At least all the classes in Lamaze breathing weren't a waste of time. Go ahead and hyperventilate through the next skid to a stop. Now take deep breaths—you've been incident-free for a week.

I will breathe.

41.

It Takes Two to Fight

Getting along with men isn't what's truly important. The vital knowledge is how to get along with a man, one man.

—PHYLLIS MCGINLEY

It seems that whenever my husband and I disagree about something, he avoids the topic of discussion and focuses on some aspect of my personality that he dislikes, and then I in turn bring up something I dislike about him," said Deb. "Pretty soon we are both hurt, angry, and frustrated—and the original disagreement hasn't even been addressed. We seem to get into this mean cycle whenever we disagree, and it's tearing our relationship apart."

No relationship is without disagreement of some kind. It is how we deal with the arguments and the value we place on not damaging each other with our words or actions that determine whether a relationship will survive and thrive or wither and die. My husband taught me this lesson. In the middle of a heated discussion that I was determined to win no matter what, he said, "I value you more than I do being right, so let's stop arguing about this." His words stopped me dead in my tracks. There was nothing more to say—I'd won. I was actually in the wrong, but I'd had a bad day and was using the argument to blow off steam.

Relationship is truly a dance, and within that dance there are opportunities to step aside and take another look at how we act and then change the steps we take, even if we've been doing the same dance all of our lives. When an argument goes in this old direction and one person steps out of the dance for even a second, as my husband did, it changes the rhythm—and it can change everything.

Today I will be the person who shifts the
emotional energy toward compassion.

42

They Need You Now

If you don't make a total commitment to whatever you're doing, then you start looking to bail out the first time the boat starts leaking. It's tough enough getting that boat to shore with everybody rowing, let alone when someone stands up and starts putting his life jacket on.

—LOU HOLTZ

It was Tuesday night, the one night I focus on self-development by attending a class. I'd spent the day catching up after a whirlwind weekend trip looking at college campuses with my daughter. I turned off my computer at 3:00 p.m. in preparation for kids returning from school, made snacks, and then sat down to begin the usual hour or so of homework. Before I left for class that night, I had to make dinner, take Troy to the dentist, and pick up Rhett from football practice.

As usual, I had everything planned and scheduled to the minute, so when the dentist appointment started fifteen minutes late I knew I was in trouble. We rushed off to football pickup, but Rhett was nowhere to be found—the team had been dismissed twenty minutes early. By the time I was headed home to drop the boys off and whip up dinner, it was obvious that I would need to call my daughter for backup. Since my kids have lived in chaos all their lives—there are so many of them, with varied schedules—this scene of switching cars and meeting at remote locations on the spur of the moment is a common occurrence. My daughter dropped what she was doing and drove to my rescue.

I was in a bad mood. All I wanted to do was go to my class, leave my family life behind for a few hours, and immerse myself in something of interest to me. I knew the class had already started by the time we exchanged the boys, but I was determined to go anyway—until I got back on the freeway and found that the traffic was at a standstill. Three exits later I got off, turned around, and headed home.

All the way home I tried to work with my anger and disappointment, to move toward acceptance of how life just *is* when you have kids. It was for the best: the kids were hungry, I hadn't found time to make dinner, everyone would benefit from my returning home, and at least they'd all go to bed on time. I sat in the driveway for a moment, took a few deep breaths, and then repeated the words that always seem to calm me: "This is your life now. It won't always be like this; they won't always need you. For this moment they come first." I walked through the door and started cooking.

There will come a time in my life when I can
do whatever I want all day long.

43.

Stranger at the Door

Guard well within yourself that treasure, kindness. Know how to give without hesitation, how to lose without regret, how to acquire without meanness.

—GEORGE SAND

It was early evening with ten minutes to spare until dinner was ready. I was out in the driveway playing basketball with my son when a young lady walked up the driveway selling magazines. She told me that she had run away from home at fourteen and was now living in a group home for girls; with these magazine sales she was trying to better her life. We talked until I heard the kitchen buzzer signaling that the chicken was cooked; I asked about her family, why she ran away, what she wanted to do with her life. She told me that all of my neighbors said they didn't want to buy anything and quickly shut the door. Then she asked me why I cared enough to listen.

I told her that seven years ago maybe I would have shut the door too. At that point in my life I was married with four healthy kids, living in a wonderful neighborhood in a big new house, with little to worry about—I would have seen her as an annoying salesperson.

Then came a move out of the country in an attempt to save my marriage, a son being diagnosed with autism, divorce—and in the end moving myself and four kids into a studio apartment off of a friend's garage. I qualified for welfare but couldn't bring myself to collect it, had not worked since college, and couldn't think past how to survive the next day.

I wasn't so different from the girl standing in my driveway. I knew what it felt like to lose everything and have to start over—and had it meant keeping a roof over my kids' heads, I would have sold magazines too. It's easy to go through our lives judging others, feeling we have nothing in common, and sure that those who live in a state of wealth, health, or lifestyle different from ours are human beings to be feared or avoided.

Until we find ourselves walking a similar path. Then we understand and are forever blessed by the knowledge of how alike all human beings are.

Acceptance of others brings me connection and joy.
Judgment brings separation.

44

Money Love

> Our deepest fear is not that we are inadequate. Our deepest fear is that we are powerful beyond measure. It is our light, not our darkness, that most frightens us.

> **—NELSON MANDELA**

I've decided no matter what the income, we all have financial stress," said Patty. "I have friends who are rich by my standards who can't pay their bills any better than I can. On top of that, when I take time to actually think about my relationship with money, I can see that I hate everything about it—but the spending."

Financial stress is a part of most people's lives; in 80 percent of divorces, finances are listed as a significant issue. A friend of mine once told me that people usually draw into their lives the things they love. She believed that I was struggling with money because I didn't love it and in fact was pushing it out of my life. "I know I'm not the only one who hates budgeting and resents paying bills," I said.

But just for the fun of it, I decided to test her hypothesis and asked myself what it would look like if I loved money, if I made an effort to shift my attitude toward it and pull it into my life instead of pushing it away. If I started to believe certain things about myself—I spend my money wisely and I'm a creative money generator—would those things actually happen, as she said they would?

I did know one thing for sure—all the time I spent worrying about money was not creating more wealth. So for one complete month I decided that every time I felt the urge to worry about money I would change my self-talk to, "I love money. I can create all the money I need."

A peaceful, stress-free month passed. My financial situation actually improved, even though I wasn't micromanaging it. More amazing than that, however, was that my relationship with money shifted drastically. Money no longer scared me; it lost its power to darken my days. I even started writing "Thank You" on the bottom of all my checks, out of gratitude that I had the money to pay for others' services.

*Loving money is okay. I can't give money away
to help others unless I have it.*

45.

One Honest Voice

Cautious, careful people, always casting about to preserve their reputations, can never effect a reform.

—SUSAN B. ANTHONY

It isn't always easy to say how you feel. Sometimes going along with the group opinion brings an already complicated mom's life one step closer to peaceful. Silence is definitely the path of least resistance, and sometimes it's the right choice. But often it's just the easiest option.

"I hate it when my teenage daughter starts pushing me to get her way," said Tina. "She is so convincing that sometimes I start doubting my own beliefs. I know how I feel, I may even have a strong opinion, but I don't feel like arguing. And when I do choose to voice my thoughts, it doesn't seem to influence how she sees it. So why bother?"

"My best friend had a run-in with the principal at our children's school," Sara said. "She was trying to get a group of parents together, who also had had negative experiences with the principal, to attend a school board meeting. I wanted to support her but felt uncomfortable. I still had two kids in the school, while her youngest was graduating and would be leaving no matter what happened to the principal. I ended up going to the meeting because it was easier than explaining how I felt."

"I was totally against the war and thought about attending the antiwar demonstrations, but I didn't want to waste my weekend when I knew that demonstrating wouldn't make any difference—we were already at war," said Brenda.

Don't ever underestimate the power of one person's heartfelt truth. The goal is not always to make something happen or to convince someone to believe as you do. Sometimes the sole purpose is to move others to thoughtful consideration. One honest, true, and passionate voice has the power to drown out a crowd. Your family, friends, and community need to hear you—even when you think they may not agree.

I choose to express my thoughts, ideas, opinions,
and beliefs so that my voice can be heard.

46

Moments of Suffering

The truth that many people never understand, until it is too
late, is that the more you try to avoid suffering the more you
suffer, because smaller and more insignificant things begin
to torture you in proportion to your fear of being hurt.

—THOMAS MERTON

In our community prayers were said, pleas were made, and
tears flowed as we said good-bye to a young man who
enlisted in the reserves a year ago. His mother holds on tight, not
knowing what tomorrow might bring; her visible suffering causes
those who look on to weep. All of us have suffered in some
way—suffering is a part of our lives as much as the joyful, celebrated moments of love, birth, or unexpected good fortune.

None of us welcomes suffering with open arms—how can we
when we already know the cost and see no benefit? Many of us just
breathe a sigh of relief that at this moment the suffering isn't
happening to us. And yet there is much we can learn through
difficulty. Those who suffer can become more open to the pain in
others, more in tune with life, grateful to have what they have, and
not so attached to what they thought they needed from their lives.

With all that's to be gained, I guess we should learn to welcome suffering with a "bring it on" attitude, banking on the
knowledge that the end result of our efforts will bring us to a

more loving, self-realized, humane space. But suffering is hard. We can't plan for it, because it just happens—most of the time we don't even see it coming before it knocks us completely off balance. So how can we prepare?

We can consciously accept the fact that things *are* going to happen no matter what we do. Then we take a leap of faith and trust that we can and will get through whatever suffering comes our way. We'll grow stronger and more human in the process, able to open our lives and hearts to others. Maybe we can't honestly say, "Bring it on," but we can say, "I will survive this pain."

The moments of suffering that life offers have as much
to teach me as moments of great joy.

47.

Ask for Help

What do we live for if not to make life less difficult for each other?

—GEORGE ELIOT

Moms are the first to offer help—to bring dinner to a neighbor who is sick or volunteer to drive a friend to the airport—but asking for help for yourself is another story.

You know the feeling of wanting to help a woman who you know is struggling with something in her life—or perhaps just struggling with two toddlers and a baby while she tries to grocery-shop! But you don't want to be nosy or draw attention to the fact that you've noticed that someone might need help. You're waiting to be asked—in the same way your friends and family are waiting to be asked to help you.

All people have visions of what they want their lives to be. It might be as simple as having an hour to yourself each night when no child needs you, or it might be committing your life to feeding the hungry. Maybe your dream is to start a new career, learn a new skill like oil painting, or mend a family relationship. Whatever it is, it's likely that you'd be able to move one step closer to your dream with help from someone.

Think about it. It would be easier to get that hour to yourself each night or the time to volunteer if your family or friends actually knew what you were trying to achieve. Unless you voice your desires and let someone know what you're trying to create and what kind of help you need, the vision you have stays locked inside your own heart.

I know that asking is hard. I had to do it recently: I asked the women who belong to my single-mother community to help me distribute information. It took me months to get the courage to send out that request by e-mail. As the responses poured in, I sat at my computer in awe, sometimes with tears in my eyes. I was reminded that at the times when we think we are most alone there is often an army of family and friends (and sometimes even people we've never met) out there just waiting to be called on. All we have to do is *ask*.

I will find my vision, voice my dreams, and ask for help, knowing that others will come to my aid.

48.

Grateful Optimism

Walk on a rainbow trail,
Walk on a trail of song,
And all about you will be beauty.
There is a way out of every dark mist,
Over a rainbow trail.

—NAVAJO SONG

Sixteen years ago I had one baby and my grandmother was visiting. I'd been complaining to her about how tired I was and how much more difficult mothering was than I had thought it would be. With each comment from her, I seemed to have a dark response. She began by telling me that my daughter was beautiful and healthy, to which I replied, "Healthy enough to have me running nonstop all day!"

When she'd had enough of my complaining, she sat me down and said, "It is easy to be happy in good times. It is easy to have faith when all is going well, and it is easy to be thankful when there is no challenge or crisis in your life. But the truth is that life was not meant to be easy." Then she continued her knitting. A few hours later, when I was carrying my screaming daughter, trying to calm her, she had more to say as she prepared a cup of tea. "I'm seventy-five years old, and in all my life I've known only three truly happy people. They all had miserable lives by your standard, but what was remarkable about them was that they were grateful anyway."

We've all heard some version of this idea—that grateful people are happy. Personally, I think I complain more than I celebrate. I let my problems rather than my triumphs dictate my thoughts, and I look at my children's futures with fear instead of with faith that within their generation lies knowledge and strength to create great change. On the other hand, I'd describe myself as a hope-filled, positive, creative person who is willing to give whatever it takes to create a better world. Within me lie both of these women—the pessimistic complainer and the grateful optimist.

I missed the simplicity of my grandmother's idea back then, but today I get it. All I need to do is be grateful for all I am and have right now, and everything else will shift into place and my view of life will change. Even when I want to throw breakfast out the window and crawl back into bed, I try to remember that it is one's view that determines happiness, and it can be created with one grateful thought at a time.

I will try to face each moment of my day with a grateful heart.

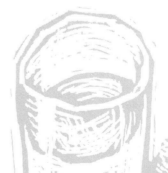

49.

What Children Remember

I do not want the peace which passes understanding, I
want the understanding which brings peace.

—HELEN KELLER

Have you ever thought about all the little things you do
every day to care for your children and what they might
remember about their lives when they grow up? Emily was at a
family function. In response to her complaint that she had no
time for herself, Emily's mom made the suggestion that she
would have more time each morning if she didn't cook whatever
her kids wanted for breakfast.

"We were debating the importance of bacon and eggs versus
a box of cereal left on the table when my brother spoke up,"
Emily said. "My brother reminded my mother that she had also
been the family short-order cook on school mornings, dishing up
waffles, pancakes, sausages, and hot chocolate. He then told my
mom that one of his fondest childhood memories was those
breakfasts. My mom never knew—not until that moment when
my thirty-eight-year-old brother told her that to this day when
he smells oatmeal he remembers sitting in the family kitchen on

those cold winter mornings, the laughter in my mom's voice, and the feeling that he was loved."

I remember my mother waking me up on a weekday morning and telling me we were going skiing instead of going to school. I can still taste the frozen candy bar I ate while she held my hand and led me back to the pool for an afternoon swim. I see her sitting by my bed while I burned the picture of the first boy who broke my heart.

The thing is, we may never know what little things we do as moms that might create a memory in our children's hearts. Maybe we do things for our children because we want to spend time with them or we want to send them off to school with a full memory of home. There may be times when we think that our efforts are a waste of time—that nobody even notices our efforts. We may not feel appreciated or receive that thank-you we're waiting to hear. But we keep doing the little things anyway—perhaps because we know that today's effort becomes tomorrow's tradition and possibly a lifelong memory.

Every day is a chance to create experiences
my children will remember.

50

A Ministry of Presence

To give without reward, or any notice, has a special quality of its own.

—ANNE MORROW LINDBERGH

Recently, my pastor told a story of one psychologist who volunteered to help in whatever way she was needed after the tragedy of September 11. This psychologist was assigned to go from one place to another within organizations like the police, airport security, and port authority to offer counseling or help to anyone who asked. For many days, whenever the counselor entered a room, the people would leave the lounge or turn up the TV so they wouldn't have to talk. She could see that people were in pain, but there was nothing she could do when their body language so clearly shut her out. Soon this psychologist was questioning why she was there at all since nobody seemed to want her. She began repeating to herself these words: "ministry of presence."

There have been many times when I have seen my children in pain, when I've heard about a situation that was a tragedy in their life or knew intuitively that they needed my help, and yet they didn't ask for my help. Saying I was nosy, they turned up the TV or left the room, telling me they could handle it. Any opinion, suggestion, or support was rejected. "A ministry of presence"—those four reassuring words—accurately describes what I offer my children hundreds of times each year. And yet, until the pastor pointed out the value of just being there ready to assist, I had relegated many of my failed attempts to help my children to a pile labeled "not good enough."

Maybe one day, while I sit stewing, knowing that I have something to offer, the moment I've been waiting for will happen. Until then, I've thrown out my old measuring stick, which calculated my success by how quickly I could fix a situation, and replaced it with a card above my computer that reads, "ministry of presence." Simply showing up has healing power, even when we cannot erase the pain, change the situation, or explain why. When our children can count on our presence day in and day out, that in itself is a ministry of love that is invaluable.

My life is a ministry of presence.

51.

You're a Safety Net

One of the oldest human needs is having someone to wonder where you are when you don't come home at night.

—MARGARET MEAD

A few times every year I take a business trip. The last time I left, only a few mishaps occurred, including my son Rhett getting eleven stitches in his forearm. The message from my husband went something like this: "Hi, I'm at Stanford Hospital in the emergency room with Rhett this time. He was spiking a ball during a volleyball game, and there was a screw sticking out of the pole. It's pretty deep, we can see almost to the bone. Sorry, I can't leave my cell phone on in the hospital. We'll call you when we're done."

Rhett called hours later to tell me that all was well. This was followed by a phone call from my daughter Brooke, who reminded me that nobody has ever been injured while I'm at home. She took her time recalling every accident, starting when her leg was run over by our babysitter when she was three, the lawn mower incident that required thirty stitches in her foot, the cut lips and eyebrows, the bike crashes, the skateboard slips—the list went on for a while.

I couldn't decide whether she was trying to make me feel guilty, insinuating that somehow my absence created the accidents, or making the point that she felt safer when I was around. Maybe my kids simply make better decisions knowing I'll be waiting for their explanation when they walk through the door. And when Mom's away, the kids will play.

But I know how my daughter feels. Even though I'm forty-three years old, I still feel more confident, protected, and less afraid when my mom is around. I think moms have some sort of shielding mechanism, perhaps a sixth sense, that allows us to call at just the right moment, or maybe it is the never-ending love energy that pours forth that helps a child believe he or she is safe. Moms can walk into an emergency situation radiating strength and a healing focus that many doctors fail to match. Whatever it is, I like the idea of being a safety net. It's nice to know that when I do need to leave home, my children miss me!

At all times I am a healing, supportive force
in the lives of my children.

52.

Create Community

The community stagnates without the impulse of the individual. The impulse dies away without the sympathy of the community.

—WILLIAM JAMES

On a recent Monday, the mother of my son's best friend died of cancer. For months the community had rallied around this family, taking the kids on weekends, bringing meals to their home, reaching out to help. It was the mothers who coordinated these efforts.

By Wednesday the end-of-the-year class parties had begun. One was a pool party for the entire sixth grade given by a mom who is constantly giving, setting up school events and offering to do all she can to create wonderful experiences for kids. She had her assistants (other mothers and fathers) on hand dishing out the ice cream, making sure nobody drowned, and taking pictures. There were many other parties, some at parks, others at community centers. Mothers coordinated these efforts as well.

On Friday I attended the funeral. As I sat in the synagogue and contemplated the sadness I felt for the children and family of this mother who died too young, I was filled with hope as I looked into the faces of the community sitting around me. Together we all stood behind the family, still wishing to comfort them.

We live in a cycle in which the challenges, experiences, successes, and losses keep marching on whether we are ready or not. What makes it all worth celebrating, as well as what gets us through the grief, is the community that stands beside us.

Mothers work very hard to create community; we do much of the planning, the reaching out, the supporting of families in need as we help our children, teachers, coaches, friends, and neighbors in whatever ways we can. Sometimes we downplay just how much we do, saying that it is nothing: "I was making dinner anyway," "The party was easy," "I was driving that direction; it was no problem taking the team." We take for granted the incredible gift we give to others every time we say yes!

I will celebrate the many ways in which I create and support community—without me, the world would be a very different place.

53.

Decisions That Hurt

Never grow a wishbone, daughter, where your backbone ought to be.

—CLEMENTINE PADDLEFORD

As mothers, we are constantly making decisions for our children, our family, and ourselves. Some of these decisions are obvious; others live in our hearts and heads for days and sometimes for months without being arrived at. Many of these decisions have lasting consequences: Should I move my father into a care facility? Should I get a divorce? Should I switch my child's school district? We go through each perceived outcome in our minds, and after enough time, whatever we might decide looks almost the same. Our intuition tells us one thing—perhaps the right direction to go—but then our heart won't allow us to go there. We've been over the good and bad points so many times that they have lost their power to convince us. One minute we're sure, but the next minute we're afraid of all the what-ifs we've come up against.

"We just found out our family dog has bone cancer," Amanda shared. "We've been told that if we amputate his leg, he has a chance of living at least six months, and maybe for many years. If we don't amputate, we'll need to put him to sleep as soon as possible.

"One moment I tell myself that he's eight years old, has had a fabulous life, and should be put to sleep without going through a traumatic surgery. On the other hand, if I had a guarantee that he would live for another few years, I'd definitely go ahead with the amputation. I feel very upset. There is no clear answer."

The operative word in that sentence is "guarantee." Decisions would be so much easier to make if we had the power to see into the future and observe the results of our decisions. But we don't have that power; often all we have to go on are the possible scenarios we've constructed in our mind.

Think of the most difficult decisions you've made. If you had had only yourself to consider, the choices would have been much easier. We feel selfish, however, if we ask, "What would be easiest, best, and most convenient for me? What do I want?" No big decision is easy—especially one that may cause someone pain—but as a mother, you have the right to consider yourself when deciding. This is not selfish; rather, it is a way to honor and support yourself as much as you do others.

I will consider myself whenever I make a decision.

54.

Emotional Self-defense

You may have to fight a battle more than once to win it.

—MARGARET THATCHER

There are all sorts of classes that teach a woman how to defend herself in case of physical attack, but there seems to be little information on emotional self-defense. This concept came to my attention around the time my daughter turned thirteen—along with the idea that perhaps there should be a parental abuse hotline!

I can deal with the usual "I hate you, you're the worst mother" statements, but when it comes to dealing with dark moods infiltrating the house—that's another thing altogether. Especially with kids these days, who are trained in the psycho lingo used to produce parental guilt.

"So you're saying I shouldn't say how I feel," she responds when I ask her to go to her room until she can be less destructive with her comments. Or, "You do think I'm fat, don't you?" when

I tell her to stop snacking so close to dinner. And it isn't just teenage children who bring out the feeling of being emotionally battered. There are bosses, friends, and spouses who use this approach in everyday interactions.

I admit that I absorb this negative energy more than most—whatever energy the other person has projected seems to go directly to my heart, where it instantly has an effect on how I feel—that is, I did until the day I learned some emotional self-defense from a friend. She told me to think of an object that I could see clearly in my mind. I chose a rose. She then told me to place the image of the rose between myself and the person who was spewing out negative comments or destructive energy. I was to then picture everything that person said going directly into the rose instead of reaching me. Then every few minutes I was to visualize the rose blowing up along with all the words that had been said. Using this strategy, I would be able to hear everything that was being said, but I would also have a protective barrier.

I thought this sounded too easy to actually work. But when I tried it, I found that I could block words in the same way physical self-defense classes teach you to block punches—by putting a barrier in the way.

Protecting myself from negative energy, thoughts,
and words that enter my life is a priority.

55

Practice Forgiveness

Holding on to anger, resentment, and hurt only gives you tense muscles, a headache, and a sore jaw from clenching your teeth. Forgiveness gives you back the laughter and the lightness in your life.

—JOAN LUNDEN

I've learned that to forgive is not to condone someone's behavior," Bridgett said. "I chose to forgive my ex-husband for hitting me the day I decided I no longer wanted that act of violence to be part of my life. For a long time I couldn't forgive him—he hurt me, ruined our marriage and the life I'd dreamed of. What I found was that as long as I couldn't forgive him, we remained oddly attached in a painful blame cycle. His behavior was my excuse for not moving forward with my own life. I wanted out of that cycle, so I released him and his actions with an act of forgiveness. It was for me, not for him. I will never understand or accept his behavior, but I've chosen to forgive him and in doing so to release myself."

Not forgiving someone, continuing to hold him accountable, keeps us stuck and unable to move on. It gives us an excuse for why we can't reach our goals or create the relationships and the life we want. Forgiving others may be very difficult, but living with the resentment and anger is sure to prolong the emotional damage. Many women look back and tear themselves down with a myriad of negative images, thoughts, and explanations—with no healing direction in mind. This keeps us stuck in the muck of our lives. Maybe you were raised by an alcoholic whose behavior scarred your childhood, and that's the reason you're a perfectionist, or depressed, or obsessive-compulsive. There's nothing you can do about it—the damage is done, right? Maybe, but forgiveness has the power to shift behaviors, thoughts, and even lifelong patterns if you focus on the goal of letting go and moving forward in your life.

Loving ourselves also requires forgiveness. We must be open to accepting our mistakes and examining the dark parts of our lives, acknowledging the choices we've made as part of our past. Your desire to move on will win the battle over past regret if you give it a chance.

I have the power to forgive right now in this moment.

56.

Grateful for Grief

Instead of looking at life as a narrowing funnel, we can see it ever widening to choose the things we want to do, to take the wisdoms we've learned and create something.

—LIZ CARPENTER

When my oldest child left for college, I thought I was ready—but no amount of anticipation could have prepared me for the empty space I found in all of the places she filled for so many years of my life. Seven years ago I went through a divorce—then I grieved the loss of a relationship and person I'd loved. Years before that, when my youngest son was diagnosed with autism, I had met grief for the first time and begun to understand that grief comes in many forms.

As mothers, we grieve in small ways throughout our lives. Most often our society talks about grief when someone dies, but we also grieve when what we hoped for ceases to be possible, when people we love move away, when a job we've depended on disappears, or when a child moves into a new stage. If we are totally honest with ourselves, it is grief we experience when the life we dreamed of in our youth proves harder to achieve than we'd thought, when our child doesn't accomplish something we'd hoped for, when a friend lets us down—and the list goes on.

Now I know that grief isn't something I can make disappear forever, so I've decided to get comfortable with it, to welcome the feelings when they decide to pop in for a visit. I embrace grief with the knowledge that only by loving someone or experiencing something with our whole hearts do we grieve the loss of that person or experience. There is no way to prepare. I want to hold my daughter, to see her smiling eyes and hear about her day. But I've allowed new thoughts to weave their way through my sadness—thoughts of gratitude that I have people, places, events, and experiences in my life that have made a difference. They have shaped and possessed me so deeply that I feel their loss— and that knowledge brings me great joy.

Grief reminds me to be grateful for the people, experiences, and events in my life that have touched me.

57.

We Are the Champions

Remember, Ginger Rogers did everything Fred Astaire did, but she did it backwards and in high heels.

—FAITH WHITTLESEY

I may not be able to win the Boston Marathon or make an Olympic rowing team, and I'll never have a poster boasting my physique. But how many of those athletes can open mail while talking on the phone? Or make dinner while correcting an English essay?" said Jamie. "I can create gourmet bag lunches and breakfast at the same time while putting on makeup and finding that special pair of lost shoes! And I do it all with the stopwatch running and the kids complaining."

We are the champions! Sing that to yourself while you're jogging down the hallway for a forgotten sweatshirt on your way to grab your briefcase and head out the door. Or on days when you're sure you aren't going to make it to the grocery store and then home to make dinner without falling asleep. Remember— life is a workout, and only the strong survive!

You might be thinking, We may be the champions, but what if we'd rather not have all of those jobs? We can do it, but what if we don't like it? Basically, if you're a mother, you may be stuck. Of course, you can do your best to ease your life's responsibilities and duties by getting rid of as many of them as possible. Or you can claim your power, use it, and celebrate it. You're doing it, you are holding your life and family together—and that accomplishment should be front-page news.

I am a champion mother, the head coach, star player, and cheerleader on my own team.

58.

A Sexy Attitude

Don't be afraid to try something new. An amateur built the Ark. Professionals built the *Titanic*.

—ANONYMOUS

always thought that men's sexual attraction was based on how a woman's body looked, that a woman needed to at least be somewhat in shape to be attractive—right? While writing an article on how men view sex, I had the pleasure of learning that nine out of ten men said they prefer a woman who obviously enjoys and loves her body, even if she is overweight, over a woman with a perfect body who constantly points out her faults or stays wrapped up in a sheet so as not to be seen after making love.

So in the end, attitude wins out over beauty! The men went on to say that the biggest turn-on is a woman who obviously enjoys sex—which is hard to do if all you can focus on is your stretch marks! The truth is that they won't see the stretch marks or cellulite unless you point them out—and there should be no time for that if you decide to embrace this sex-crazed attitude that men seem to crave.

We all like the idea, but the challenge for most of us is that our behavior patterns are hard to change, even if we know that a change of attitude would turn our man on. There's more to it than desire. We may be self-conscious, or perhaps we've disliked our body for so long that it's too hard simply to drop the sheets and run naked around the bed. It isn't just our men who crave a sexually free woman—we long to feel this freedom as well. We may just not know how.

Truth be told, there is no easy way to begin. You just have to jump in with the belief that you are one sexy woman who is capable of fully enjoying her body and participating in sex with an open, inviting attitude. You may want to have a little "let's start our sex life over again" talk with your partner so that you don't cause a heart attack at the first unveiling of the new you. Tell him you are game to try this new approach and that you hope he will support you in exploring your sexuality. Yes, ladies, this is a learn-by-doing event.

I will not wait for someone else to create a sexy mindset—
I will create it myself.

59

PMS =
Perfectly Made System

In all things of nature there is something of the marvelous.

—ARISTOTLE

W hen my daughter first got her period, I tried to create a celebratory mood," said Jane. "I congratulated her on becoming a woman, told her how blessed and lucky she was to have a healthy body, one that could now bear children. She glared at me and said, 'Yippee! Like I want children. What I really want is to put off this bleeding thing for at least ten years. Is there a pill for that?' before stomping off to her room and closing the door.

"So much for the whole joy of becoming a woman thing, I thought, a little discouraged, believing I'd failed to make this a happy, remembered event for both mother and daughter. But then I started thinking about menstruation and how our whole society deals with it. When a woman is moody, men make comments about how she must be having her period or, worse, 'be on the rag.' Then there is the whole PMS thing—which labels the body's natural reaction to changing hormone levels as a syndrome that needs to be treated with drugs.

"I do realize there are severe symptoms related to menstruation, but in general I think that women would feel much better about the whole process if as a society we viewed it differently.

Just think back to the days when women left the village to be alone when they had their periods—sign me up for that! Personally, all my mood swings would disappear entirely if I had four days of solitude each month.

"No wonder my daughter glared at me," Jane concluded. "We no longer dress our girls in white robes, braid their hair, give them gifts, and surround them with wise women to celebrate this new stage of life. There is no female initiation ceremony in our Western society that reminds all of us that the natural world of the moon, earth, and stars miraculously follows the same thirty-day cycle as our bodies. We've become so out of touch, demanding that our bodies feel balanced every day when being out of balance is our natural state."

*When my period arrives, I will take a day of solitude
and notice what happens to my PMS.*

60.

Demon Days

There is no pleasure in having nothing to do; the fun is in having lots to do and not doing it.

—MARY LITTLE

I think it's funny when my friends pretend they never have days when things are completely out of control," said Julia. "It happens to me regularly. I get up and my kids won't do their jobs; some animal has died in my yard and I have to figure out what to do with it. Then I sit down to work and can't get motivated, so I head for the box of chocolates I've hidden (so that I won't be tempted to eat them). I call these kinds of days Demon Days.

"When I was younger, I'd just say that I had a bad day, or that I couldn't get anything to go right—but now when I see a Demon Day coming, I just sit back and head for the chocolates right away. I pull out a good book or turn on a favorite movie, because I figure, what's the point in fighting it? I allow myself the freedom to feel how I feel, and do what I want to do. The next day I seem to wake up refreshed and recharged, ready to take on the world."

We focus a lot of energy on getting stuff done. Most of us can muddle through a long to-do list even on the worst of days. But if we can't for some reason, we feel very discouraged, depressed, or frustrated at how behind we have become.

We are afraid to give in to a bad day, throw in the towel, have a sense of humor about it, and just say, "Oh well, time for a nap!" We've learned to disconnect our feelings, push through a workday, and complete the chores our children forgot to do, regardless of how we feel.

You will feel more empowered if you learn to wave the white surrender flag and do what Julia did—declare a Demon Day. It doesn't matter how you choose to spend this day; even if you have to go into work, the point is to accept that this is a day when nothing of any great significance is going to be accomplished—and you don't care!

P.S. Every mother needs a box of chocolates hidden where nobody can find them.

The next time a bad day comes my way,
I'm going to take a step back—and enjoy it!

61

To Tempt or Not to Tempt

Woman is the peg on which the wit hangs his jest, the preacher his text, the cynic his grouch, and the sinner his justification.

—HELEN ROWLAND

Eve offered Adam the apple, the girl with the short skirt tempted the man into a sexual advance. . . . I'm tired of the idea of woman as the temptress. Why aren't we talking instead about men's lack of self-control?" asked Brenda.

"My daughter was actually told by an administrator at her school that the dress code was put into effect because one of the male teachers was charged with sexual misconduct—and the way the girl dressed was partly to blame! A naked man could stand in front of me and I wouldn't assault him—would you?"

This whole idea of woman as temptress lives in our collective consciousness with both positive and negative consequences. Women, especially mothers with daughters, are constantly thinking about what kind of message we are sending. We're bombarded by images of sexy, beautiful women, and part of us wants that—we want to feel sensual, attractive, and desired. But we seem to be caught somewhere in the middle. Should I wear the low-cut top because it's the right color and I like the way it looks—or would someone get the wrong idea?

On the other hand, we want to be free from this constraint and allowed to express ourselves in any way we want without the fear that some man—a friend, teacher, or neighbor—will misinterpret our intent.

In many ways this same concept was the message of the women's movement: let us be who we are—give us equal rights, equal laws, and an equal right to choose what we want. The women won—we do get to choose—but now it is up to us to free ourselves from the idea that sexual expression is a bad thing.

Don't be afraid to be a woman. Swing those hips, wear what you want, spray on a little perfume—embrace the female power that's yours, guilt-free.

It's time to shake free of my guilt, remove the word "fault" from my vocabulary, and claim my life and sexuality with a passion.

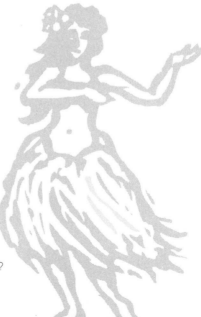

62

Body Connection

Challenges make you discover things about yourself that you never really knew. They're what make the instrument stretch—what make you go beyond the norm.

—CICELY TYSON

Why is it that everything experts say will make me feel good takes so much work?" Angela asked. "I know that exercise is important, but trying to schedule it into my life is such a pain. When I actually get to the gym or go for a run, I don't really enjoy it. Plus, if I'm going to schedule time away from my kids and get a babysitter, I want to be doing something totally relaxing—not sweating on a treadmill!"

There are women who swear by exercise as a way to increase energy, decrease mood issues like depression, and promote sounder sleep patterns. But maybe you're more like Angela, a woman who hasn't found a form of exercise that calls out to her and offers a way to connect with her physically active body in an inspiring, playful way.

If you could just shift your view of exercise slightly and define it as time to connect and play with your body, maybe an inspiring idea would come to your mind. It probably isn't that you don't like to move—after all, you move all day long. Rather, it might be that you can't find time to move in the structured way that exercise has been defined in the past.

Maybe you've never taken the time to ask yourself what kind of physical activity you'd actually like to do or learn. Maybe you were never taught to swim as a kid, or never took a karate class. Maybe your family would not think of social dance as exercise, so you've never considered signing up for that Friday night class.

Or maybe you haven't given yourself the freedom to create space for physical activity in your life on your own terms. Walking with a friend, biking to the store with your child, and dancing while doing the dishes do count as movement, and if you vary the daily "exercise" activity, it may become a joy instead of a burden.

The bottom line is that mothers need a way to connect with their bodies, to nurture them, move with them, and enjoy growing stronger.

I will discover more ways to play—to connect
with and nurture my body.

63

Age-old Obsession

Age is something that doesn't matter, unless you are a cheese.

—BILLIE BURKE

I remember the day my mom told me that she felt she'd become invisible to the world," said Samantha. "I thought she'd lost her mind, until she explained herself. She said that all her life she had taken great care to look beautiful, to stay in shape, and to choose her clothing in order to draw attention from onlookers. Until one day when my sister and I were in our late twenties, and she noticed that no matter how good she looked, she wasn't turning the heads she once did—men and women had stopped looking at her. At first she was devastated, but then she started to think of the benefits that might go along with this new stage of her life.

"'Imagine what I can do with all the extra time I used to spend beautifying myself,' Mom had said with a chuckle. Of course, I thought she was kidding herself, that she would never be able to get past her desire to be beautiful. But she did, and the results were astounding. She took up painting, joined a women's choir, had weekly teas with lady friends in her garden, and felt what she called a sense of great relief at finally being content with herself."

It is never too early for women to embrace the benefits of aging. So much of our lives seem to be lived on the treadmill of anti-aging strategies, from creams to surgery—anything to stop the process. How much more fulfilling life might be if we learned to accept our body's natural process of aging and to see it as an opportunity to focus our attention on other, more interesting, areas of life.

Of course, to welcome the reality of aging doesn't mean you have to look sloppy and stop dying your hair or whatever else makes you feel good. It simply means that you stop stressing out about the fact that you're getting older.

Remember—you have to buy into the social definition of beauty, age, and what a woman should or could be in order for that definition to have an impact on your life. The choice is always yours—and that choice may determine whether you live depressed and afraid or open and jubilant. Choose wisely.

I have a choice to celebrate all the ages and stages of my life.

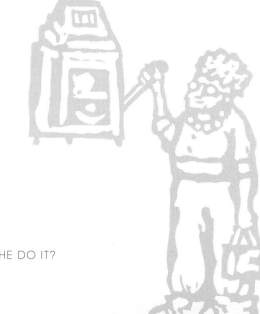

64.

Surround Yourself with Beauty

Think of all the beauty still left around you and be happy.

—ANNE FRANK

My friend Carol gave me an aromatherapy candle as a gift," said Terri. "It was an expensive one with decorative paper describing the ingredients wrapped around the center and then tied with a velvet bow. Carol knows that when I buy candles I usually go for the plain, on sale, or inexpensive variety!

"I set the candle next to my bed and decided to light it as I read that night before falling asleep. In moments my room was filled with the scent of lavender. My mood shifted and lightened as I thoroughly enjoyed the beauty of that candle. When I woke in the morning, I was inspired to clean off my dresser and straighten up my room. Afterward I called Carol to thank her for a gift that had reminded me that beauty has the power to inspire." Before this experience, Terri said, she used to laugh at magazine cover claims that changing your environment could change your mood.

The next week she bought one beautiful flowered teacup from an antique store and decided that she would use it every time she sat down for a cup of tea. She then created one small space in her garden where she could sit. She planted a few flowers around her chair. This is where she sits to drink her tea from her antique cup each morning. Too often we believe that adding beauty to our lives involves remodeling an entire room in our home, completely overhauling a garden patch, or buying a new wardrobe—so we give up before we begin. Or we settle for five cheap candles instead of buying the one we really want. What Carol taught Terri with her gift was that the smallest object of beauty can transform a space if it draws our attention, even for a moment, toward a smile, a feeling of gratitude, or a sense of wonder.

I will find a thing of beauty and give it to a friend.

65.

Things Kids Say

Little boy to his dad: "You remember I asked you the other night how much is a million dollars?"

"Yes," answered the dad.

"Well, Dad, 'a hell of a lot of money' isn't the real answer."

—ANONYMOUS

There seems to be nothing that makes me quite as happy as *order*. I experience the joy of cleaning out my office every six months. During one of those cleaning binges, I ran across an old writing journal titled "Things the Kids Say." I opened it and found myself laughing at each entry as I remembered *exactly* the moment the words were spoken, what the kids looked like, even how I felt.

I wish I'd written more. One was a conversation I had with my then-six-year-old son. I told him that his smile was magical, and he said, "I don't pack my smile everywhere I go. It's not going to be on that airplane to New Zealand." Even at six, Rhett had a way of basically staying on topic and still getting his bigger point across! Another time I was walking with my four-year-old son on a paved hiking trail when he lay down in the middle of the trail on the only piece of shade we'd seen. I gave him a few seconds to enjoy the cool ground, but when I saw an oncoming group of walkers, I asked him to get up. He said, "I was here first; if I get up they'll take my place." I remember how entertained I was by my children's innocent ideas, wit, humor, and understanding of the world even at the earliest ages. I know you've all heard this before, but that moment could have been a month ago, and today my sons are both almost grown up. Thousands of these moments fill our mothering lives.

Today my goal is to look into the faces of my teenagers and allow myself to embrace the moment, to be as entertained by who they are today as I was when they were young children. And I'm going to keep that journal out and write more so I can laugh with the memories of their teen years in my old age.

I will be present to my children today, open to their goodness, humor, and uniqueness.

66.

Grow a Friendship

It's always been my feeling that God lends you your children until they're about eighteen years old. If you haven't made your points with them by then, it's too late.

—BETTY FORD

With three sisters, two daughters, and currently six children in my home who are teenagers, I understand the teen years and the love-hate relationship that most mothers and daughters seem to go through. I've learned to cherish the moments when my seventeen-year-old daughter, Wesley, wants to be with me and dismiss the moments when she doesn't—without feeling hurt or rejected.

Recently I attended a water polo tournament with Wesley. She was sitting with her team with a towel over her head to stay out of the sun. A few minutes later, to my surprise, she left her team and came to sit next to me. Then she did something she hasn't done in public since she was eight. She asked if she could lie down and put her head in my lap. She let me stroke her hair as we talked about her feelings about the game she had just played. We talked with the ease of lifelong loving friends. All of this in clear view of her team, her coaches, and other parents!

I was flooded with the knowledge that nothing is as precious or as strong as the mother-child bond. No matter how many times they push you away, there will be a moment in time when you've let go enough and they've grown up enough that the conflict can cease and the friendship can begin. It's a glorious moment, one that is worth the work, understanding, and love it takes to raise a child. When that moment comes, celebrate it.

Even when my children push me away,
they need my love and understanding.

67.

Never Forget Your Girlfriends

It is the friends that you can call at 4:00 a.m. that matter.

—MARLENE DIETRICH

There is something about sharing the past with a friend that cannot be duplicated with friendships in later years. After all, receiving your first kiss, getting your period, and graduating from high school happen only once.

It seems to be the old friends who can write or call anytime and still have something to talk about, even if you have to resort to, "Remember the time we stole your dad's cigarettes and smoked them with those guys down by the creek?" The conversation inevitably leads first to laughter at the shared memory and then to an outpouring of where you are in your lives now—the joy and struggles you face. Through an old friend's eyes, you get a clear glimpse of who you are—and who you were before this grown-up life as a mother took over!

I don't have as much time these days to develop friendships. Sometimes I'm just too lazy to try, or I feel that it takes too much time away from my kids and busy life to really get to know someone. We'd have to start at the beginning and fill in so many gaps—is it worth the effort, I wonder? Then I have to remind myself that the women I get to know today might be the friends of twenty years when I turn sixty—and isn't this stage just as interesting and full of challenges as my younger years? I want friends in my life who are present the day my daughter graduates from high school or my first grandchild is born. That means I need to create memories and adventures with new friends that can be shared ten years from now.

As I look back on my life, it has always been my girlfriends who have sustained and supported me—laughing, crying, scheming, accepting, encouraging, and loving me—without asking or expecting me to be anything but myself. No matter how busy our mothering lives get, we cannot forget that our friends are a gift—bringing us joy, lightening our load with their presence, and inspiring us to value ourselves.

I am blessed to have friends who love and
accept me exactly as I am.

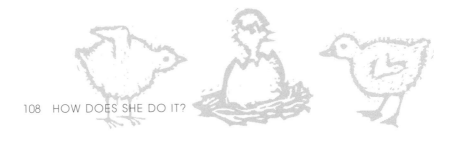

68.

Fitting In

Each person grows not only by her own talents and development of her inner beliefs, but also by what she receives from the persons around her.

—IRIS HABERLI

My son started seventh grade at a new school where all of the boys wore their shorts halfway down their butts with boxer underwear," Jill laughed. "I made it very clear to my son from the beginning that he would not dress like those boys.

"A few weeks into the school year my son came home obviously upset. He said that he felt completely out of place and hadn't made any friends because he dressed so preppy—and it was my fault! I told him that this was just the beginning, that if he compromised what he wanted now, what would he do when the peer group was telling him he wasn't cool unless he tried drugs or other things? I want him to learn how to stand up to people and be who he is, not what they want him to be."

We have the difficult job of encouraging children to be original, to make their own choices and become strong enough to stand alone—and at the same time helping them find ways to fit in.

If we are honest, we all want to fit into our community, to be valued and acknowledged. So it isn't hard to understand that our children express the desire to be part of a peer group of their own, to be accepted and included. That doesn't mean they do anything asked of them just to be liked, but it can mean buying your kid a pair of pants you hate, allowing your daughter to pierce her belly button, or indulging whatever other trendy choice the group has made.

Think past the outward appearance and support the small, insignificant requests even when you wish your child would choose otherwise. By accepting the fact that your child wants to be part of a group and will take actions to be like the group no matter what you do, you can focus your energy and attention on the bigger and more important choices—like drugs, drinking, violence, stealing, and sex. We need to pick our battles wisely and be willing to compromise on the ones that in the long run make no difference at all.

I understand my child's need to fit in, and I will offer support and guidance according to my intuitive wisdom.

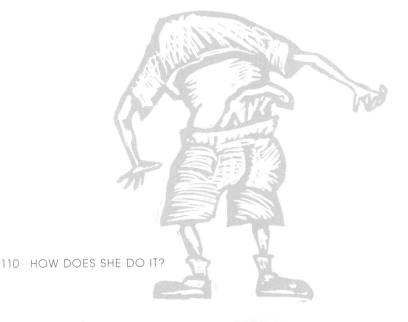

69.

Kids Who
Challenge Life

A mother is neither cocky nor proud, because she knows
the school principal may call at any minute to report that
her child has just driven a motorcycle through the gym-
nasium.

—MARY KAY BLAKELY

I signed my son up for a jazz music camp, thinking that if he
loved to play drums for his rock band, surely he'd love to
learn jazz drumming techniques. After the first day he was
threatening to start a fight just to get kicked out of camp—he
hated it. When the performance came at the end of the week, he
refused to play.

Needless to say, I was incredibly disappointed. My expec-
tation that this camp would awaken a passion for jazz in him
fizzled. I wanted to force him to play and tried to make him feel
guilty by pointing out how he was letting down the other kids in
his ensemble. He was visibly distraught but simply repeated over
and over, "I'm not playing."

As hard as it feels sometimes, we need to give those we love—
our children, family, and friends—space to experience life on their
own terms. We need to stand back and allow the consequences to

play themselves out, without considering our expectations. Each time we step in and override their decision, it sends a clear message that we don't trust them to be in charge of their own lives.

I ended up telling my son that I trusted him to have thought through the consequences of his decision *and* that I believed in his ability to manage his own life. However, he would need to take responsibility and confront the head of the music camp himself with his explanation for why he wouldn't play. He did, and then we drove home.

In the same way, as women, we need to be in charge of our own growth and happiness. When we truly believe we can handle our own lives, that we are competent to make our own decisions and have the right to private spaces, the feeling of self-confidence and competence grows. Self-respect as well as mutual respect flourishes. Within every loving relationship there needs to be space for each person to determine who he or she is and what he or she wants. In the end we are all individually responsible for the person we grow into.

I am in charge of my own life, my own decisions,
and my own growth.

70.

Negotiation–
Our Specialty

The thing women have got to learn is that nobody gives
you power. You Just take it.

—ROSEANNE BARR

Halloween is a good example of a mother's bargaining and
negotiating power. Boys especially seem to walk into the
costume store and immediately point out the bloodiest and scari-
est masks. We cringe at the thought of teachers or neighbors seeing our innocent eight-year-old with a knife through his head.

But we know that some agreement has to be reached, so we
throw out the first negotiating point—"There will be no
weapons sticking out of the body"—to which our son protests.
We say nothing. Time passes, and as each costume is suggested
we say (of the ones we would refuse to buy), "That would be
okay, but didn't so-and-so wear it last year?" Most of the time, if
we are passive for long enough, our son gets tired of shopping
and settles for something we can live with. This give-and-take is
an art that mothers excel at—knowing when to offer this or
when to accept that to finalize a deal.

This skill develops over time, as does the courage to stand
our ground, which will be a key skill when the adolescent years

arrive! What began at seven or eight as an argument over a Halloween costume is now a major debate over curfews, body piercing, and friends. Being passive no longer works—instead, we have to really listen so that we can use our minds to strategize a plan we want to negotiate toward.

In all cases, we teach our children important life skills as we model our willingness to negotiate. The first is that we can't always have things the way we want them. We have to be willing to listen to another's point of view, and we need to listen with an open mind. When we hear a good point, we need to acknowledge it fully, giving our child credit for coming up with an idea that helps the negotiation process continue. In turn, the goal is to create a relationship in which our child will also listen and acknowledge good points.

*I will listen with an open mind and use
my negotiation skills wisely.*

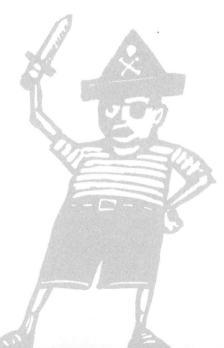

71

Space to Grow

You don't have to be afraid of change. You don't have to worry about what's been taken away. Just look to see what's been added.

—JACKIE GREER

I've had many chances in my life to practice letting go. I guess it's getting easier—it's supposed to anyway! Somehow holding on to the known feels much easier than letting go or having to welcome the unknown. Often letting go brings with it a gut-wrenching "Why me?" or "Why this?" or "Why now?"

Last week our family dog was very ill. I had to choose between letting him live medicated and in pain or putting him to sleep. I chose to put him to sleep. He had a disease I couldn't fix. I sat on the floor of our veterinarian's office, trying to let him go, yet holding on as he left this world peacefully.

We decorate our homes and then move, make good friends and then have to say good-bye. We start and lose jobs, birth children and then send them on to lives of their own. We love deeply until death forces us to let go. It seems that learning how to let go of all we've worked to create is one of the biggest challenges that life presents.

There are benefits: we can begin to discover the space that is created in our lives every time we are able to release something or someone. We can give ourselves choices: now that X has happened, I'll have time for A, B, or C. We can ask new questions: "How do I want to fill this space or time?" In the end the gift we receive when we finally let go is the expansion of our hearts—we make room for new experiences as well as the memories that live on.

My life is in a constant state of growth, which includes
some things dying, while others are germinating.
I will embrace this cycle with anticipation.

72.

Embrace Your Strength

We deceive ourselves when we fancy that only weakness needs support. Strength needs it far more.

—MADAME SWETCHINE

Not long ago I was giving a workshop for single mothers. We came to the exercise where I ask each woman to think of one object that represents a strength she has. I gave a few examples: a rubber band for flexibility, a blank piece of paper for the ability to create something from nothing, a pretty stone to represent the ability to be appealing and strong at the same time. At first there was silence. Then Joan spoke up. "I'm so used to thinking about all my weaknesses and the things I want to improve upon that I never think of myself as someone with strengths."

Many women sitting there that day nodded their heads in agreement. I wondered what kept all these women focused on what they were lacking instead of celebrating what they had.

We pushed ahead with the exercise until everyone had thought of one object. As each woman announced her object and the strength that belonged to her, I could see smiles begin to form on all of their faces.

No matter what challenge we face in our lives, we sell ourselves short when we focus on our limitations rather than on how to best use all of our strengths. To use the strengths we have, we need to know about them. That means spending time identifying what they are and then practicing them each day. It means taking the compliments we receive from others and embracing our character strengths as more important, valuable, and usable in our lives than all the aspects of ourselves we wish we could improve on.

Think of three objects that represent three of your strengths. If possible, collect these objects and put them someplace where you'll see them every day. Each time you look upon them, remind yourself that these strengths belong to you.

Know that your strengths are at your disposal. They sit in your back pocket waiting—tools to be used as you grow and become the woman you want to be.

When I am feeling weak, I will remember my strengths.

73.

Food for Thought

I've been on a diet for two weeks and all I've lost is two weeks.

—TOTIE FIELDS

I spent some time this weekend contemplating the relationship that women have with food. It is pretty funny if you think about it: we crave it, hate it, are led astray by it, indulge in it, fast from it, set limits with it, and swoon in ecstasy over it. Sounds like an almost human relationship to me.

You can also learn a lot about a woman's life, about the way she sets goals, and about how she sees herself by the way she approaches food. One woman looks guilty, fills her plate with a few bites of each food, and then pushes the food from side to side before covering the remaining food with a pile of salt so she won't be tempted to finish it off. Another woman seems to take what she wants, salivates over every morsel, and indulges with a big appreciative smile. In those images may be a clue to the communal psyche of women. Some of us believe that we can't really stuff our faces with food (or with life) or we might get too plump, that we need to sacrifice, push things aside, and refrain from indulging to become the woman society expects us to be.

We all know that food is more than nourishment, that it is reward, celebration, and sometimes addiction. It fills us and gives us something to look forward to—even to obsess about when we'd rather not face other things in our life. Considering how many women talk about diets and how many articles focus on body improvement, I'm willing to bet that few of us have thought about our own personal relationship with food in a positive way. Nor do we take time to examine the delicacies of life that, like our food, we may crave but set aside and cover with salt.

I had a conversation with my sixteen-year-old daughter on this topic. She made the startling comment that "daughters would not have eating disorders, think they were fat, or struggle with enjoying food if their own mothers liked and appreciated their own bodies more." That's a thought that we as mothers might want to consider and perhaps act on.

When we sit down to a meal, what are we communicating? Not good enough, more sacrifice needed, don't enjoy anything too much, you don't want to be caught stuffing your face! Food is just the tip of the iceberg, but it does have a story to tell us about our personal beliefs—a story worth listening to.

I will fill my stomach and life with delicacies I enjoy.

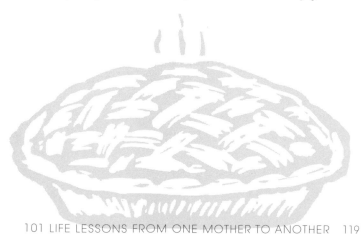

74.

Learning to "See Funny"

No life is so hard that you can't make it easier by the way you take it.

—ELLEN GLASGOW

I f you've ever said, "We are going to laugh about this down the road!" why not seize the moment and start laughing immediately? If you are expecting to be frustrated or stressed, then you probably will be and you won't be able to see anything funny. I usually choose the stressed-out route. I certainly wasn't laughing when I pulled a gas hose out of the pump and then drove for twenty feet before noticing—even though the children in the backseat were practically choking back tears they were laughing so hard.

Nor was I laughing when the pan of lasagna I stuck in the oven at four o'clock, with a huge note giving instructions for someone to take it out of the oven, was still in the oven burned to a crisp at ten when I returned home—and nobody smelled it!

You may choose—as I have many times in the past—to sulk, scream, or complain about the unfairness of the situation, convinced that someone has a voodoo doll made in your likeness. Or you can ask yourself, "How could this situation be worse?" Use your imagination, ladies, and you may begin to understand what it means to "see funny"! When it feels like you are experiencing one of those stories that will be told for years to come as a source of family entertainment, find a way to laugh in the moment. Concentrate on seeing funny—when you think about it, even the difficulties in life can be pretty humorous if you are looking to be entertained.

Today, as difficulties present themselves,
I will use humor to diffuse the tension.

75.

Sensuality Discovered

It's never too late—in fiction or in life—to revise.

—NANCY THAYER

Too rushed to sip a cup of tea, pick a flower, light a candle, or listen to soothing music? Has it been years since you took a bubble bath, repainted your bedroom, or bought a pair of silk underwear? You may be neglecting your sensual soul and in doing so depriving yourself of a woman's most treasured instinctual ability—to connect with the sights, sounds, touch, and smell of life.

"We bought a new house five years ago," said Bridgett. "For the first three years I had hopes of remodeling, so I did nothing to our bedroom. It was freezing in the winter, with wood floors and no carpeting. The bed was pushed into a corner, so I slept hitting the wall, and those walls were made of redwood, which gave the whole room the appearance of a cave. One night, as I slipped under my expensive high-thread-count cotton sheets, I experienced a flash of insight.

"I hated my bedroom. There was nothing in it that made me want to make love or even sit and read a book. I never thought about how my home environment might be affecting my mood—until I was lying there surrounded by ugly things.

"I hatched a new plan—I was going to rearrange that room. It literally took a weekend. I ordered carpet to cover the wood floor, painted the walls, went to a used furniture store to buy a four-post bed frame, which I painted the same color as the walls, and purchased aromatherapy candles on sale, along with a new bedspread. The place was transformed—and it was much cheaper than the therapy I was headed for!"

Sometimes we forget that we are sensual beings who need to wear silk underwear—even if it is underneath sweatpants.

I will blossom today by choosing to surround myself with beauty.

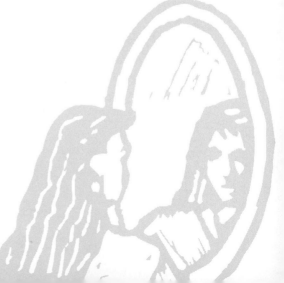

76

Mirror, Mirror

How many cares one loses when one decides not to be
something, but to be someone.

— COCO CHANEL

Every so often, while doing my regular nightly regimen
of washing my face, I stop to really look into my own
eyes," said Gloria, the mother of two college-age children. "I'm
never sure what prompts this shift from looking at myself to
looking into myself, but the moment it happens is always unpre-
dictable and profound. I find myself saying, 'Oh, there you are,'
followed by, 'Is that really me?' I look different—older, more
stressed, less enlightened, unfamiliar, and vulnerable.

"In this moment a blank, expressionless woman stares back at
me. Where is the pleasant face that smiles while putting makeup
on? Or the disappointed woman who wished for another outcome?

"I take a moment to look into my eyes, which spend so much
time lovingly looking into the eyes of others, and consciously give
back to myself the same look of acceptance, love, and acknowledgment that I so easily give. For just that moment in the bathroom mirror, I connect with myself. I take a moment to really see
inside, to touch the lifelines, to look without judgment, to
embrace without question the woman that I am. I'm still in there,
that girl who has grown into an older woman with wrinkles."

There is much to be learned by accepting the fact that behind the daily masks we wear of mother, wife, and friend is a woman who may sometimes be out of touch with her essence—an emerging soul just waiting to be heard. We take so little time out of our lives to look into our own eyes, to ask ourselves a question. No matter how much time we spend living in the world or with our family, children, and jobs, we are still in there, waiting for a moment with ourselves.

Today I will look into my own eyes with love and acceptance.

77.

Mom's Yearly Bonus

Too many people are ready to carry the stool when the piano needs to be moved.

—ANONYMOUS

Happy Labor Day to all of you who labor hard and long every minute of the year. I'm not sure if mothers are included in the group who have been given this holiday—but if we aren't, I think we should be added! When I went through the divorce process, my soon-to-be-ex-husband said to his attorney—in front of me—that it would have been cheaper to hire a maid, cook, surrogate mother, and babysitter than it had been to marry me.

I went home and added up one month's worth of what it would have cost him to hire someone in my place. My four kids were all under ten at the time. I can still remember the grin on his attorney's face when I presented my list the next day and he realized that the cost to hire me would have taken practically his entire income that year.

Most of us know that our services are undervalued—but we also know that what we bring to our families is more precious than anything we strive to gain materially in our lives. After all, why do we go to work in the first place? To take care of the people we love and to see them grow into responsible, caring, honest, and creative adults.

The hand that rocks the cradle rules the world. I don't remember who said that, but it makes perfect sense because love is the greatest motivator, and that can't be taught in business school or on the job no matter how much money you make. It is taught by mothers, given freely even though there is no real bonus to look forward to, or paid vacation, or acknowledgment of the importance of a job well done.

So let this moment of praise be the certificate, the gold watch, the year-end bonus. We as mothers *know* the job we've done, and we're *grateful*, because without our joint efforts and contributions, the world would be a very different place.

P.S. However, a real gold watch every once in a while wouldn't be so bad!

I will celebrate all that I do each day with the knowledge that my contribution is of great significance.

78.

Shop Till You Drop

When you have only two pennies left in the world, buy a loaf of bread with one and a lily with the other.

—CHINESE PROVERB

I admit it: I hate shopping for groceries, kids' clothes, or household items, but I love shopping for me. Walking from shop to shop, looking at anything from clothes to furniture, all by myself with no time limit—that's what puts me in an elated meditative state. It may actually be the only time I spend thinking solely about what I want or like. Nobody is asking me questions, wanting something from me, or demanding my attention.

I can wander from rack to rack, feel the textures, delight in the colors, and imagine myself reviving my wardrobe. Or I can explore an arts and crafts store and take note of unusual projects I might attempt in the months to come. So I asked myself, if I enjoy this time of self-attention so much, why haven't I done it more often? Why do I hide what I've purchased, sometimes for months, so my husband and kids won't notice that I've bought something new? The answer was that I had long felt guilty about shopping. Like many women, I believed that shopping is a waste of time as well as a temptation to spend money that I can't really afford to spend.

I told a girlfriend of my dilemma. She shared with me the secret of her self-care fund, an account into which she puts part of the budgeted household money every month so that she has something for herself. Nobody knows about this account. For the first year she said she found very little extra money to put into it. Then, when she paid attention to how much money was spent on each of her kids every month, she decided to cut their spending in half and put that money into her fund.

If you think about it, women have been shoppers since the beginning of time. We carried our baskets out into the wilderness to gather whatever caught our eye. We'd bring our findings back to the cave, weave them into clothing, or create tasty meals. The enjoyment of touching, feeling, draping ourselves in beautiful things, and being curious about the new and unusual is inborn. We need to claim this right and enjoy it for what it is—a way to nurture ourselves. We all deserve a self-care account so we can splurge on self-indulgence once in a while!

I have the right to spend money on myself.

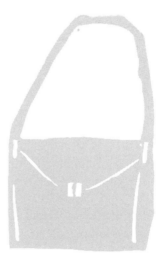

79

Peaceful Existence

We are apt to mistake our vocation by looking out of the
way for occasions to exercise great and rare virtues, and
by stepping over the ordinary ones that lie directly in the
road before us.

—HANNAH MORE

I have been delivered into a state of peaceful existence. For
more days than in any other period of my life, I've had time
to myself. I haven't had to make dinners or pack lunches, and on
some days my car has not even left the garage. I've been able to
stock the refrigerator with all the foods I like to eat, go for walks
with friends, and run errands at a relaxed pace instead of at warp
speed—I haven't had to rush to get back in time for something.
Amazing what kind of thoughts this independence and self-
indulgence can create. I like this lifestyle—and I plan to find a
way to bring some of this peace and attention to my own needs
into my life when all the kids return in a few days.

I've talked to my boys while they're at their dad's house.
They're making their own breakfasts and lunches and spending
part of each day watching TV. At first I felt at a loss—I wanted to
demand that their father do what I do, that he feed them, follow
my rules, and supply more directed activity. After letting me
vent, one of my wise friends suggested that the boys would be
fine and that I desperately needed a break. She told me to let it

go, to not think about what they were doing, to trust that they would be safe, and to totally enjoy myself.

So here I sit with only a few days left before the house is full again—I feel like a changed woman. Perhaps I do more than I need to do for my children. They are surviving fine without me, without all my little pieces of advice, without my waffles or eggs and bacon for breakfast each morning, and watching TV hasn't killed all of their brain cells. So I'm asking myself, can I survive without doing so much for them? Can I keep up this newfound self-love and attention in the face of the daily mothering responsibility that's so familiar to me? We'll see.

There are many things my children can and will do for themselves—if I let them.

80.

If Moms Ruled the World

To the world you might be just one person, but to one person you just might be the world.

—ANONYMOUS

Martin Luther King Jr. lives on. I see him in the faces of people protesting war, his message written across thousands of signs. As mothers, we have a unique view of war that policymakers will never understand: it is our children who will be sent to the front lines. I've often thought that if every nation's leaders would step aside for just thirty days and let the women of their country meet with the women of the warring neighbor, peace would be reached.

Maybe that is too simplistic, but how do we as women teach our children to be peacemakers in a world where adult leaders are not using their "words" (as we've taught our children) but rather their "fists"? The model of conflict resolution we use in our homes and in our schools—to sit together, list the problems, and then brainstorm solutions that everyone can agree to try—is it just a theory?

I'm asking myself today, how can I use what is happening in our world right now to teach and inform my children? How can I model peace and take a stand that will help my children feel that they can make a difference, even in a world that seems to be spiraling out of control?

It may seem an overwhelming task, and yet I believe that mothers are the most important teachers. We can take small personal steps toward tolerance in our lives and choices. We can model open-minded questioning followed by intelligent ideas for solutions. We can be ready to take action when action needs to be taken, whether that be in giving food to our homeless, mediating peaceful solutions to arguments in our homes, or calling the mother of a bullying child. We can support each other as mothers as we reach out with kindness and understanding.

So when we remember Dr. King and his dream, as well as the other peacemakers of our time, may we each find within us the courage to demand peace. Each of us has to believe that it is still possible to create the world Dr. King envisioned, not just for those of us in the United States, but for everyone. With a shared vision, peace is possible.

There are things I can do today that will create
a more peaceful world.

81.

Girls' Night Out

Each friend represents a world in us, a world possibly not born until they arrive.

—ANAIS NIN

Women do things for each other. We watch children, deliver meals when someone is sick, and review possible hairstyles before a major beauty change is made. We cry with each other when something bad happens, and we celebrate when something good happens.

We have to be willing to offer to others the kind of friendships we crave. If we want to have friends who will tell us that we look awful in that dress, or that we might be making a mistake, we have to be just as honest, brave, and loving toward them.

Today my best friend ended a phone conversation with these words: "Did you know that you're already way better than good enough? You're amazing." And she went on to list everything that she sees in me that I sometimes forget. I was feeling a little down when I called her, but when I hung up I remembered the woman I am—the woman she sees!

Our girlfriends cannot be treated as an afterthought—as something to fit into our lives after everyone else's needs have been written on the family calendar. We *need* the support, nurturing, and self-expression our gal pals allow. The time we spend engrossed in conversation, figuring out our lives, complaining about our partners, crying over a loss, or celebrating a great achievement is medicine to our souls—it heals us and releases us from the everyday responsibilities we have as mothers.

Friends allow us to be truly ourselves. We don't have to dress them, do their homework, or pay for their education—we can just show up and enjoy. Open your heart to the women in your life. Take a chance and tell a woman you feel drawn to that you'd like to know her better. Plan a girls' night out once a month. Send your best friend from high school a letter telling her what you loved about your friendship—even if you haven't talked to her in ten years. Schedule an afternoon tea for your girlfriends and *buy* cookies—it doesn't matter!

I will enjoy the gift of having friends!

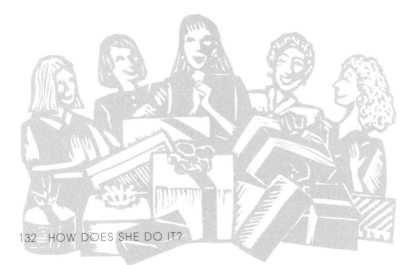

82

A Time to Give

You don't pay back your parents. You can't. The debt you owe them gets collected by your children, who hand it down in turn. It's a sort of entailment.

—LOIS McMASTER BUJOLD

This is the third day I've spent flat on my back sick in bed. I'm a frustrated patient who instead of resting thinks of everything that isn't getting done. Three of my children are sick as well. The good news is that they are old enough to medicate themselves and have decided as a group that I'm the worst off, so nobody has asked me to do anything but make one pot of cream of wheat cereal (after their failed attempt that resembled glue).

The last time I was in bed for three days I was ten years old. My mom made sick days special. She would wheel a TV into my room and serve me meals of my choice. She even taught me how to knit mittens and slippers so I wouldn't be bored. My mom seemed happy to have me home, or at least I never felt that my being sick was putting her out. I also remember how it was when she was sick. The house was dark, and it felt like someone had taken a straw and sucked the energy out of our home.

I don't remember anyone making her meals and bringing them to her in bed. I guess we all thought it was enough to let her sleep. There are so many things in life you don't really think about or truly appreciate until the tables are turned. Now I totally understand my mother's frustration when she would make her way to the kitchen for something to eat and find it a total mess. We'd ask if she was better yet as we lounged on the couch.

One day when I was complaining about my kids not helping me, my mom told me that there is not enough time in a life for a child to pay back a mother for all the minutes spent loving and caring. The way it works is that you give the time, love, and energy back to your own kids in a cycle of caregiving. I guess that is why, when I'm feeling sick, down, or in need of nurturing, I still want my mother. What a lifelong gift of love mothers are to their children.

The gift I received from my mother—to give even when I'm tired or sick—is the gift I now give to my children.

83.

I Think I Can

If you think you can, you can. And if you think you can't, you're right.

—MARY KAY ASH

There are two children's books I keep in my office, *The Little Engine That Could,* and *The Giving Tree.* With these two wise stories in hand, I feel ready to face most of the challenges that come my way.

The Little Engine That Could is the story of a train who, to make it up a big hill, keeps chanting, "I think I can, I think I can." Many of us get stuck on the steep hills of our lives simply because we impose limitations based on what we believe about ourselves. We say, "I can't do it." And there we sit, afraid to push on, worried that our weaknesses might be discovered, and sure that if we risk taking the brakes off we might actually roll backward.

I've often told my children that whenever someone asks if I can do something—anything—I say yes, and then I figure out how to do it later. That is what the little train taught me—to say I can and then deal with the consequences. When I'm afraid of failing, I actually say these words under my breath with great conviction—"I can do this!"

The Giving Tree is a story about a tree who loved a boy and so gave the boy anything he asked for until all the tree had left was a stump. At first reading I thought, how stupid of the tree—that tree needs to learn how to say no! Then I got it—the story wasn't exactly about the tree. The tree was happy no matter what, but the boy who got everything he asked for was never happy—he just kept wanting more. The tree, even though it lost every limb, didn't really lose anything, because it gave its love freely.

With these concepts close to my heart, I don't need to read any other self-help books to reach a state of happiness. All I need to do is learn to be content with what I have, give out of a feeling of love instead of guilt, and believe that I can do whatever I set my mind to doing. Pretty simple ideas—that's why we teach them to children. The problem is that sometimes as adults we forget how simple life could be.

I can do anything I set my mind to—I am an amazing woman.

84

The Spectacular Lives Inside Each of Us

Aerodynamically, the bumblebee shouldn't be able to fly, but the bumblebee doesn't know it, so it goes on flying anyway.

—MARY KAY ASH

Before my eldest daughter graduated from high school, my father and I took her out to lunch. We began talking about college, and he asked her what she thought she might want to study. Her ideas ranged from being an art curator to working in public relations, or maybe radio or TV broadcasting. In the end she came to the conclusion that she didn't really know.

I've had enough talks with my daughter to know that one of her concerns in choosing a career is making enough money to support the life she wants. But I also know that she wants to find work she's passionate about. In her words, "Who wants to wake up each day and do something they don't like just for money?" Already the struggle between responsibility and self-fulfillment has begun!

Her eighteen years of life experience have not yet taught her a truth that has taken years of living for me to understand—the spectacular lives inside each of us. It is alive through the passions we have, whether they be painting, poetry, cooking, dancing, writing press releases, or whatever brings spark to our lives. The spectacular lives within our talents and special gifts. These we can bring to any job if we look hard enough for ways to express them. Even to the jobs we feel stuck with!

I look into my daughter's eyes and realize that I don't need to be concerned with what field she studies, as long as she's willing to study herself. If she looks within to find her passions, talents, and gifts, and if she's willing to bring those with her to whatever moment in life she's faced with, she will find great success as well as fulfillment.

As her mother, my job is not over. She will leave my home to begin a new chapter in her life, but I am still her guide. I know what she has not yet learned, and I'm ready for the challenging task at hand—to continue the study of myself—for we cannot teach our children what we have not learned ourselves.

I will bring my passion and talents to whatever job I do.

85.

Me First

The greatest danger for most of us is not that our aim is too high and we miss it, but that it is too low and we reach it.

—MICHELANGELO

We spend so many years of our lives wanting to be some-body. Then somewhere around age thirty-five we begin to see that maybe we should have been more specific about who or what we wanted to be! Maybe we had an idea at one point, but then life stepped in our way—children were born, we had responsibilities to consider. Somehow the clear vision of what we wanted was set aside.

How do we rediscover what we want and allow ourselves the opportunity to dream—not just the small dreams but the big ones? Is it possible to go for what we really want while also maintaining the life we already have? I think it is—*if* we claim the right to put ourselves first at least some of the time.

There is a saying I hear my son and his friends use all the time: "First is the worst, second is the best!" Usually it is the person who has lost who begins this chant. Still, we've been raised in a society where the words "Me first" have very negative connotations. "Self-sacrifice" is listed first on a mother's job description, followed by "compassionate," "nurturing," and "wise." Rarely on that list do we find the words "aggressive," "determined," "self-promoting," or "driven." Maybe we need to write new definitions for ourselves to include all these words—perhaps we don't have to be one or the other.

It's time we abolish the "them first" attitude that we've become so accustomed to regarding our children, homes, and spouses. Me first! Say it loud and clear. Say it right now without one flicker of guilt. Now go out and make it a reality—put yourself first a few times every day. Get into the practice of asking yourself, "What do I want?" before you commit to something your child or spouse wants.

I claim my right to put myself first at least some of the time.

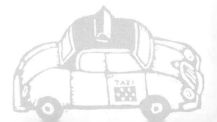

86.

Taxi Service

We're always being told that time is running out; it is, but getting things done won't stop it.

—JOAN SILBER

There is nothing a mother can do about car duty. I've often thought that I could have learned a new career or earned a Ph.D. with all those hours I've spent driving. Each week, after I added up the time spent behind the wheel, I would say: "Just think of what I could be doing with that time—reading a book, taking a yoga class, or taking a nap!"

My resentment was rooted in the belief that this was wasted time—that it was just service to them and of no value to me. To shift my mindset and create new behaviors during car time, I had to set up different expectations for everyone. The new plan: we would talk with each other. We wouldn't listen to the radio or stare blankly ahead, and if asked a question, we would answer with more than three-word sentences.

During those first few car trips with the new rules in place, eyes would roll and the response would be short and choppy— but once I changed my focus, the kids shifted theirs as well. Sometimes it took a gentle reminder: when my daughter tried to make me feel guilty for not having the time to talk with her one evening, I reminded her that we had had an hour together earlier that day when she chose to say nothing. Another time I had to give a respect talk: "Out of respect for my taking time out of my day to pick you up, I expect you to take a few minutes to tell me what is going on in your life. If you are unable to do that, then I suggest you find another ride."

Now that I have two children who drive themselves, I look back on my car time with a new appreciation. My best parenting moments happened when I had just one child in the car with me. That child had my full attention, and when I felt brave enough, I brought up the difficult subjects like sex, love, drugs, and future dreams. Over time my children learned that they could trust me, that I was a good listener who was willing to hear what they had to say without correcting them. By taking part in the daily dialogue, we grew closer. I moved from resentment to gratitude.

Within inconveniences lie hidden gifts—if I
am open to receiving them.

87.

Married with Children

A great marriage is not when the "perfect couple" comes together. It is when an imperfect couple learns to enjoy their differences.

—DAVE MEURER

W hen you're having kids, everyone talks about how tired you'll be, how your life will change," said Ginger, the mother of two toddlers. "But nobody tells you that you might wake up one morning and glare with contempt at your spouse for no reason you can articulate—other than the fact that in that particular moment you hate your life, are tired of grimy hands and mornings spent digging in the sand at the park while your spouse gets to put on nice clothes, eat lunch in a restaurant, and spend the day conversing with adults!

"The exhaustion I feel dealing with the little things puts me over the edge by the end of the day. Even when I tell myself that I want to be nice, communicative, loving, and maybe even sexual toward my partner, my words sound like barking. It's like the life we had before kids—as friends, partners, and lovers—has been replaced with an endless list of issues, responsibilities, and sleepless nights."

Ginger has a point, wouldn't you agree? Keeping the love, understanding, and cooperation going when the resentment, anger, misunderstanding, and exhaustion set in can feel as challenging as climbing Mount Everest with a broken ankle. So how do we do it? How do we keep things in perspective? Will those intimate, supportive conversations we used to have be replaced with diaper rash dialogue or curfew conflicts for the rest of our child-rearing lives?

Yes—and no. Those intimate conversations can happen—they just need to be scheduled (along with sex, time off, nights out, and shared housework). You'll have to risk telling the truth and admitting that your expectations of parenting are not matching the reality. And don't expect that admitting this means anything is going to change—but how you feel is important, and your partner needs to know. You'll also need to learn how to work together and let each partner's strength support the other's weaknesses. But remember—it isn't a fair partnership if one person lists all household upkeep as a weakness!

This is the most difficult stage you will face as a couple, so give each other a break. Think of it as a real-life survivor show, and then sit back and be entertained!

Even when my expectations are not met,
I will remember that I am loved.

88.

Heal Each Other

Never doubt that a small group of thoughtful, committed citizens can change the world. Indeed, it is the only thing that ever has.

—MARGARET MEAD

A girlfriend told me about a dream she had. She was standing on the balcony of her home holding her two small children as she watched a mushroom cloud rise above San Francisco. She spoke of the horror she felt in knowing there was nothing she could do.

I hiked last week with another friend; we talked about feeling depressed, which is not an ordinary state of mind for either of us. As we talked, both of us realized that underneath the day-to-day stuff we are managing is a fear that is seeping deep into our unconscious.

As mothers, we experience world events and the threat of disaster on many different levels. As activists willing to create a world where people are created equal, valued, and given basic rights, we want to see the unjust punished. As creators of life and protectors of our children, we wish to escape to some remote location where the concepts of violence, retaliation, punishment, and war can play out far from our everyday life. So of course we are all confused, scared, and uncertain of what the coming years might bring.

How can we process the bad dreams and feelings of dread as we wait? We can send letters to our representatives, march in rallies, and wish for other countries to veto war plans. We can even hope for some kind of wisdom virus to attack the brains of our nation's leaders. But again, the outcome is out of our control.

What we can do is simply support each other—even when there are no answers to the terrifying events that happen daily. We can begin by embracing and healing each other. Then, with others by our side, we can take action, speak our minds, and remember that any effort, no matter how small, is like a small stone cast into still water. We may not make waves, but many ripples still change the look of the pond.

I will allow all the healing power I have within me
to be released into the world.

89.

A Visit to the Outhouse

People who fight fire with fire usually end up with ashes.

—ABIGAIL VAN BUREN

Have you ever noticed that your children are very different with you than they are with other people? In the past month I've heard all of the following:

- "I never have a problem getting Troy to do his homework" (said my husband while I was having a shouting match with Troy over summer reading)

- "Rhett was a joy to have with us in Hawaii. He consistently cleaned up the kitchen without being asked" (said a friend's parent, an hour after I'd grounded Rhett for leaving the dishes two nights in a row)

- "Brooke is the most amazing organizer—she completely reorganized every closet in our house this summer" (said my daughter's summer employer; every closet in my home looks like we've been hit by a tornado—including the one in Brooke's room!)

My list of these kinds of comments is endless—and consistent through each age of my children's development. I can take these comments as compliments: at least my kids know how they are supposed to act, even if they don't do it at home or for me.

What is hardest for me is having my children tell me how they feel and then to watch them act as if those negative feelings don't exist. I admit this is partly my fault—I've established myself as my children's most accessible emotional dumping area. I can sit for hours hearing how difficult my child's life is: homework is stressful; they have no friends; they're fat, ugly, unliked, unpopular, or unsuccessful; teachers pick on them; and the party they'd looked forward to was no fun.

Then, half an hour later, they'll be on the phone to a friend relaying the exact story or situation with a cheery smile, laughing and joking—while I'm still worried about the issues they've just described. In contrast, when the good times come—the first day of school, making a team they've tried out for, a first call from a boy or girl they've liked—and I ask for details, the kind of in-depth details I get regarding all the negative stuff, they respond, "You ask so many questions—it was fine!"

"It hardly seems fair," I complain to my husband. "I do all the work, put up with all the crap, and everyone else gets to enjoy them." His response: "They can't shit on you if you put the seat down!"

I experience my children's worst traits because they love and trust me most!

90.

Dropping the Ball

The thing that is really hard, and really amazing, is giving up on being perfect and beginning the work of becoming yourself.

—ANNA QUINDLEN

I sat down at my desk after being sick for two weeks and looked at a to-do list that had grown to three pages," said Jean, the mother of two toddlers. "I laughed to myself at the realization that moms are not really allowed time off from life. It all keeps on going: the kids keep eating, the clothes are still dirty, and deadlines are set at work. I looked through my long list with two questions in mind: How am I going to prioritize this? How can I make this all up this week and get back on track?"

Learning how to drop the ball, cross things off, say no, and decide what you need to do for yourself is one of the toughest life lessons. It is all about recognizing what you value most, and for most of us mothers our own names would come at the bottom of the list. It also requires a thick skin, because you have to set aside your own fear of what others might think of you.

This includes your children when you tell them you can make it to only one game this week, your friends when you cancel a standing hiking date, a teacher when you call and tell her your child can't have homework this week because you are recovering from an illness.

"I made many calls to back out of commitments, and not everyone was happy with me," said Jean. "But here I sit seven days later with no to-do list, ready to begin my week caught up and happy."

Is this a selfish approach to life? Maybe. Could we as mothers be a little more self-centered? Absolutely. I know that there are things that need to get done in our lives for our families and our work, but I challenge you today to take a really hard look at your list. Could dinner be simplified? Do you really have to take on a new project at work? Is there any task that could be dropped so as to make your life more manageable or enjoyable? Drop the ball, cross it off, or say *no*. With a little practice, a thick skin is easy to grow!

It's all right to say no when I don't want to do something.

91

Life Design 101

Advances are made by those with at least a touch of irrational confidence in what they can do.

—JOAN L. CURCIO

"When I was a teenager, I wanted to be shorter so the boys would like me," said Victoria. "Then as I grew I wanted my skin to be clearer, my breasts larger, my memory stronger. There was always something about my life I wanted to be different. I found myself looking back all the time, regretting choices I'd made or resenting all the ways my life could have been easier if only. . . .

"My aunt was visiting one day when I was around eighteen years old—she was drinking a cup of tea and chatting with my mother and me. All of a sudden she put her cup down and said, 'Victoria, would you please stop all your complaining about life? Everyone is dealt a hand, just like in cards—you have absolutely no control over the cards you get. What I want to know is, how do you plan to play the hand you've been dealt?'

"Until that moment it never dawned on me how much happier I would be working with who and what I actually was, to design the life I wanted, rather than looking backwards at what could have been or forward to what might be if only I could change X. From that day forward I started asking myself, 'What are you going to make with what you've got? Which cards are you going to play first?'"

As unfair as life might seem at times, we've each been dealt a hand that we can't give back to the dealer. Maybe that hand includes superb intelligence, creative ingenuity, the ability to serve others, beauty beyond measure, or great wealth. Maybe you hold some cards you would have passed on if given a choice, like divorce, disability, or financial struggle. The true measure of a successful life is not found by comparing the cards, so many of which are out of our control; rather, it is determined by how well we play our hand.

Today I will appreciate the cards I hold and play the hand I've been dealt with courage.

92.

Secrets to Keep

If you reveal your secrets to the wind, you should not blame the wind for revealing them to the trees.

—KAHLIL GIBRAN

Did you know you're allowed to have secrets, to hide things, to keep some part of yourself to yourself? This was news to me. For years I've been running my life with the assumption that honesty is the best policy—complete honesty when possible. All the articles I've read about how secrets damage relationships, how hiding a part of yourself can stunt emotional development and keep intimacy at bay, have scared me into submission. We live in the "let it all hang out" era—right? We tune in to talk shows and listen to women blurt out their most intimate and delicate lifelong secrets in less than three minutes.

Yet there may be aspects of who we are, what we want, and experiences we've had in our lives that we want to keep to ourselves or just leave behind. Maybe it's as simple as having a new dress hiding in our closet that we aren't ready to unveil. Maybe we played hooky from work to go to the beach. It could be something more serious, like having chosen an abortion when we were young or being insanely jealous of a best friend.

Some secrets, like abuse, drug use, alcoholism, are the dangerous kind, and it is absolutely necessary to tell them to protect yourself and your family.

But there are other secrets—choices you've made, opinions you hold right now, even negative thoughts about your spouse—that don't necessarily need to be aired. You aren't required to answer everything your kids, family, friends, or spouse ask you. There is always the polite "I'm not really ready to talk about that," or the humorous "That's a personal question—I pass," or the vague "That's a good question; I'll have to think about it."

You don't owe anyone an explanation for your choices unless those choices will hurt another person. You get to decide what part of your truth to tell and what you want to keep to yourself.

I am entitled to a private life.
What I share with others is my choice.

93

Stand-in Mom

If someone listens, or stretches out a hand, or whispers a
kind word of encouragement, or attempts to understand
a lonely person, extraordinary things begin to happen.

—LORETTA GIRZARTIS

It was three in the afternoon when I got the call. My
daughter's best friend, Julie, asked me to drive her to the
mall to pick out a dress for a dance that night. Her mother was
gone for the day. I was busy too, and feeling a little resentful that
her own mother hadn't made the time to take her shopping,"
said Grace. "I had stuff I needed to do with my own kids, but
something in this girl's pleading convinced me to say yes.

"As I sat outside the dressing room, I figured out why she had
called me. With each dress she tried on, she made a comment
about how her mother thinks she should lose a little weight, or that
her mom wouldn't really like this one. She ended by saying that her
mother refused to take her shopping because they always fought.

"Julie has a great mom—she's really involved and supportive
of Julie—but they clash miserably in this particular area. I
decided then that sometimes kids just need a stand-in mom—
someone they aren't as close to, someone who will listen and *not*
tell them what to do—and in that moment I felt happy and
proud that Julie called on me."

There are times when a child needs a mother, but none is available for one reason or another. That's when we get the chance to become a stand-in mom. It could be as simple as talking with a child who's obviously distressed or as difficult as caring for a child for months while the mother undergoes chemotherapy. Your first impression may be that this is just another responsibility to add to an already busy life, but being asked to take it on is really a great honor.

Keep your ears and heart open for the opportunity to reach out to a child whose mother can't—you'll never regret it. And if the time ever comes when you are that mother in need, someone will be there to step in for you.

*I will always have space in my life to reach out
to a child who needs me.*

94.

Digging Deep Enough

Creative minds have always been known to survive any kind of bad training.

—ANNA FREUD

I've been to three different churches in the last year, attended a meditation group, a yoga class, a Shamanism workshop, and still haven't found what I'm looking for," said Stacey, a single mother of three. "I was raised going to church each week, attending Sunday school, and saying grace before each meal, but I just haven't been able to offer that kind of spiritual stability to my children.

"I know it's a sorry excuse, but they have activities on Sunday, and sometimes I'm just too lazy to make the effort. I want some sort of spiritual life for our family—and I'm searching—but nothing feels right yet. One of my friends used the following analogy when she was trying to explain why I should stay with a spiritual practice long enough to get somewhere with it. 'Imagine digging for water in your yard. You dig each hole to about twelve inches and then go on to the next. Pretty soon your yard is covered with hundreds of holes, but none of them is deep enough to reach water.' Her point was that I hadn't dug deep enough to discover the spiritual practice that was right for me."

Mothers are the spiritual center of a family, whether we want to be or not. We teach our children about God, a greater power, values, or whatever it is that we believe in simply in the way we live our lives. Spirituality is not necessarily religion. It is wherever and however you feel connected with the universe, your internal voice, or your greater power.

Gardening can be a spiritual practice if done with awe and reverence for the natural world, with the feeling of gratefulness for the dirt, the sun, and the opportunity to embrace the earth. Driving your children, making dinner, or doing homework can be a spiritual practice if you are totally present in the moment— thankful and open to what you have to give and receive from the experience.

Sometimes we forget to stop and sink into ourselves. To dig deep into what we believe in and then find a way to express it in our daily lives. We miss the opportunity to find peace in a moment of silence, or understanding in the way a wave breaks on the sand.

In everyday moments, spirit is within me. It is my unique connection to self and the world—my gift of comfort.

95.

The Real Holiday

There are two ways of spreading light—to be the candle or the mirror that reflects it.

—EDITH WHARTON

Each year beginning about a week before Thanksgiving a feeling of dread descends upon me," said Samantha, the mother of two toddlers. "There seems to be no real reason why I should be wishing for January 1 to arrive instead of feeling the anticipation of good times to come. I have wonderful memories of the holidays and traditions I love. I also look forward to piling all the kids into the car, driving to the top of a local mountain, and trudging over field and forest to find the perfect tree. I've spent some time wondering why the holidays hold less joy for me each year. The answer comes immediately—it is the responsibility of creating it all."

Many moms feel like Samantha. The holidays take so much energy—to decorate the house, send out the cards, buy the presents, make the cookies, and adhere to the traditions the family loves. In reality, the to-do list leaves little time to sit and enjoy all that a mother works to create for her family.

So we sit with the question, what can we do about it? We could simplify things, do less, buy less, and expect less. And yet, the one thing most of us feel throughout the holiday season is a deep appreciation of family, friends, and tradition. When everyone sits joyously at the table, we feel that the effort it takes to get together and celebrate is worth it. When we look into our children's faces as they help with a community party, we understand why all the fuss: the holidays are about connection, giving, loving, and taking the time to acknowledge those who matter.

"All I need to do to enjoy instead of dread this holiday season is to be clear that I'm the one who has a vision of what I want to create, the traditions that are important to me, and the love I want to share," Samantha decided. "And then to acknowledge that creating a wonderful holiday for my family models to them exactly what Christmas is about for me—the giving of ourselves."

I am the one who gets to choose what I want to create in my life.

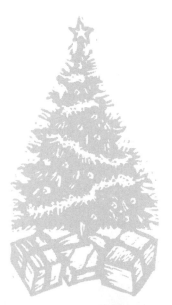

96

Romantic Interlude

Love doesn't just sit there like a stone; it has to be made,
like bread, remade all the time, made new.

—URSULA K. LE GUIN

My husband came home last night with an idea he'd
heard on the radio about how to create more romance
in our lives," said Ellen. "I'd just finished an hour of homework,
made dinner, and was starting the laundry after a long day at
work. Needless to say, I smiled a bit sarcastically at his suggestion—and then asked if there was a way to incorporate folding
the towels into his plan. Adding that, as far as I knew, romance
was not sex. Was he still interested?

"The thought of going out of my way to create romance was
a little threatening, not because we'd grown apart—because we
still talked about everything—but we had kind of grown out of
that passionate stage.

"I looked through the magazines around my house and found
romantic ideas in most of them—I guess I had skipped those sections
at first reading! One suggested I take a provocative picture of myself
and hide it in his briefcase. Then I was to call him at work, tell him
I wanted him, and hint that he might want to check his briefcase. I
laughed when I read it, thinking, who would do something like
that? The suggestion in itself produced a wave of sensuality within

me, but the doing of it seemed so out of character. Would he love it? Absolutely. But did I have the courage? I wasn't sure.

"It took a month for me to have the guts to ask my best friend to take a picture of me in lingerie—we laughed the whole time, and she ended up taking a few pictures for her boyfriend too. When I finally went through with it—of course he was floored—he drove straight home from work. What surprised me most was how much that one simple act changed the way we saw each other. I was challenged to step outside my comfort zone and focus on getting a little romance back into our lives instead of putting all my energy into the kids. He in turn looked for ways to surprise and seduce me—it was a great lift for our relationship."

With a little creative attention, I will rekindle romance in my relationship.

97.

Wild Woman

When we lose touch with the instinctive psyche, we live in a semi-destroyed state and images and powers that are natural to the feminine are not allowed full development.

—CLARISSA PINKOLA ESTES

When I hear the words "wild woman," a feeling of longing passes through me—a yearning to be wild and free, belonging to nobody but myself. In touch with my instinctive nature, like a wild seed floating on the wind looking for fertile wet earth to sink my roots into.

To me, being wild means to live in touch with my instinctual nature, to feel no shame, to jump out from behind the dark bushes of my life and stand proudly drinking from the stream of opportunities. Taking what I want, giving when I want to, and sleeping in the grass with no fences barring my escape!

But I'm not a wild animal—I'm more like a domesticated dog. All things to all people, hoping for attention and reward as I follow the expectations of my pack. Yet within me is a kinship with the wild feminine—even though I'm not quite sure how to find her. I know that I want my playful nature back. I know I need to listen more intently to my instinct and intuition than I do to the call of responsibility. I know that this wild side still exists within me, even in our tamed society.

The question is, how do we tap into this great source of feminine expression and power? How do we shed our old patterns, behaviors, and beliefs and open up the windows of our mind to new wild woman possibilities without shirking our responsibilities?

We envision ourselves as wild women, running naked, free from others' expectations, free from our homes and all they imply. We imagine what it might be like to howl at the moon or roll in the mud. We learn to laugh in the face of attack, ready to show our claws if we have to. And we listen—we always listen to the age-old feminine voice that calls us to follow our intuition.

We bring that imagery into our lives. We remember how it feels to be wet and dirty from the mud, and the earth becomes familiar to us—somehow we remember it. We demand that the fences be removed, that we be free to choose ourselves and our desires without feeling ashamed. We keep searching for the wild within us as we discover new ways to let it out.

I claim my right to be a wild woman!

98.
The Color of Your Life

If you don't like the way the world is, you change it. You have
an obligation to change it. You just do it one step at a time.

—MARIAN WRIGHT EDELMAN

One day an old friend whom I hadn't seen in nine months
called," Danielle said. "She sounded depressed, so I asked
if I could come and visit her. When I got to her apartment, I was
in shock. Everything in it was a shade of black, from the bedspread to the place mats.

"She reluctantly agreed to go and sit out on the balcony to
talk. I got right to the point and told her how worried I was. She
had many excuses: she'd been out of work, she'd broken up with
her boyfriend and just wasn't feeling very happy. This woman
used to love bright colors. She wore funky things, big earrings,
and even hats sometimes. I wondered when and why she had
made the choice to surround herself in black, without a living
plant anywhere near.

"We took a trip to a nursery to buy a few plants. On the way
back I ran into a linen store and bought a few bright sheets. I
wanted her to see that with little color splashes here and there,
as well as by opening the drapes to let the sun in, she would
begin to feel different. Back in her apartment, I pulled out the
sheets, threw one over her bed, one over her couch, and one
over her table as a tablecloth. She smiled at my parting gift. A

few days later she called to say that she felt hopeful—not exactly happy, but much better than she had been feeling."

Often our exterior landscape reflects our inner landscape— we surround ourselves with and create from our inner mood or feelings. But if this is true, it would make sense that changing the exterior should also have an effect on the interior. Painting a room, buying a colorful scarf, and planting bright flowers are not necessarily cures for depression or the blues, but they certainly will help you feel better than draping your life in black.

Look around your home, your car, your closet—your life. What are the colors that surround you? Do they express the joy you'd like to feel each day, the woman you are, the direction you're heading? If not, change the colors of your life.

I will surround myself with color, drape myself in color, and look daily for ways to brighten my life.

99.

Family Memories

Oh, to be only half as wonderful as my child thought I was when he was small, and only half as stupid as my teenager now thinks I am.

—REBECCA RICHARDS

This year we celebrated my parents' forty-fifth wedding anniversary. As I watched them together, I couldn't help but admire the fact that they were still together and loving each other. They were still choosing to spend the day alone at the beach, still having interesting conversations, and still smiling at each other with knowing glances when family stories from the past began to be told.

My kids were sitting at the table when I decided to ask my parents questions about their life together. I was glad to see my children listen intently to how my parents met (on a blind date), how the romance went, and what their wedding was like. From there the conversation moved to dating and curfews. (It's funny how every conversation moves to rules and curfews if teens are involved!) I couldn't remember coming in after curfew until my younger brother broke into the conversation with the following comment: "Hold on, have all of you forgotten that there were three little sets of eyes who saw everything you did—even things you didn't know we saw—and you definitely were not as good as you're describing?" My kids' ears perked up at that comment! We were all laughing about selective memory and how facts seem to change over time.

My brother's comments made me think. As close as I am to my parents, brothers, and sisters, and even though we lived with the same parents in the same house with basically the same upbringing, we have very different memories. The recollections seem to be a mix of what really happened, what we wish had happened, and how we've processed those experiences as adults. What casts a light of hope, fun, and continuity over all of them, good and bad, is the fact that we are still together sharing, laughing, and celebrating life with each other.

Every day I create memories within my family that bind us together and allow us to celebrate life.

100.

Time to Dance

If I had my life to live over, I would start barefoot earlier in the spring and stay that way later in the fall. I would go to more dances. I would ride more merry-go-rounds. I would pick more daisies.

—NADINE STAIR

L ife has often been described as a dance. The question is, do we join in the dance or sit it out and watch from the sidelines? Maybe we've tried to dance but had our foot stepped on, or we asked someone to join our dance just to be rejected. Maybe our dance with life up to this point has been one of anger, abuse, neglect, or sadness, so we are afraid to dance. Maybe we've come to the conclusion that it's just easier to be a wallflower. Sitting it out, there's less opportunity to fail, no risks, and few challenges.

But if we really want our lives to be our own, at some point we have to claim them. We have to become engaged in the process, ready to take our chances. It sounds easy—just stand up and walk toward the action—but the attitude we have while doing the steps listed on our dance card determines the kind of life we live.

Think about the last ballet you saw, or the last wedding you attended where you danced so hard you had blisters on your feet and your jaw muscles ached in the morning from grinning so large. Imagine moving with life in the same way—intertwined, lifted, twirled, and laughing with every part of your being engaged in self-expression. To dance with life is to be playful, engaged, and willing—very different from sitting in fear or watching in wait for the perfect moment to join in, waiting for a time when you believe you'll be ready. If you don't remember what it feels like to dance, give it a try: move your feet, flail your arms in the air, bounce up and down, giggle and shake. You'll feel an instant attitude of joyfulness, which can often be overshadowed by the day-to-day life, so full of responsibilities and things to do.

Remember this moment of freedom, this moment when you chose to dance. Remember the feeling of lightness, the laughter and joy. Let go, shake free of the old dances, the old patterns that keep you glued to a seat, afraid to set foot onto the dance floor of life.

If I invite my body to move,
my heart will have no choice but to follow.

101.

What Is Enough?

To feel valued, to know, even if only once in a while, that you can do a job well is an absolutely marvelous feeling.

—BARBARA WALTERS

We spend our lives fixing, growing, nudging, and sometimes outright pushing our children onward. I believe that my job is to notice the little things that need attention in my children's lives—social skills they may lack, learning difficulties unnoticed at school, problems on the playground, issues at home—and the list goes on. In fact, I have to admit that most of my time is spent in this frame of mind, looking for problems to fix.

I rarely give equal attention to the overall picture that is my child, the gains already made. I focus on the girls my eleven-year-old son didn't get to dance with at the first dance—instead of encouraging him to tell me about the girls he did dance with. I focus on how disappointed my daughter feels when her senior pictures didn't turn out as she had hoped, instead of looking into her eyes and reminding her how lucky she is that it was the camera that failed and not her beautiful face!

Alas, some of us worry that if we don't pick up all the pieces, we aren't doing our job. But I'm starting to believe we might have a more important job to do. And that is to model the belief to our children that who they are is enough, that not everything can or should be fixed, and that the constant desire to be better than we are and to want more than we have leads to a life in which nothing is enough. Self-esteem, belief in one's abilities, and ultimately love of self grow in all of us when the skills we already have get validated.

It's time to stop our crusade to fix and improve our children's lives and instead to start voicing our belief that who they are right now is good enough and should be celebrated.

After trying this out on my kids, I'm going to do the same for myself.

Who I am and what I have is enough.

Acknowledgments

My heartfelt thanks to all the women whose stories brighten, inspire, and bring to life the pages of this book. Many of you are part of my Internet mothering community (www.CompleteMom.com) and receive "Mothering Moments" from me each week. Your comments, support, and insight have made this book possible.

Many people working together created this book. Thanks to my agent, Al Zuckerman, and Writers House for continued support and encouragement no matter what project I propose. To the team at HarperSanFrancisco, especially my editor, Renee Sedliar, for understanding exactly what I am trying to say. To Miki Terasawa, Margery Buchanan, Kris Tobiassen, and Lisa Zuniga for the talent and effort they've brought to the creation, design, and promotion of this book.

I am continually grateful for the constant support and inspiration I draw from my family. Without my children—Wesley, Brooke, Rhett, Troy, Adam, and Eric—I would have few stories to tell. Thanks to my husband, Al, for so enthusiastically living this chaotic life alongside me as my partner and best friend. And to my parents, Dave and Nancy Maley, for being there always with love, time, and understanding.

Finally, my thanks to Julia York, my hiking partner and life-long friend, for your hours of listening. Much of my writing comes from conversations and ideas we've shared over the years. Your belief in me keeps me going.